David T. Kelly (Ed.)

Adalat®
in the Asian Pacific Region

With 44 Figures and 37 Tables

Springer-Verlag Berlin Heidelberg New York
London Paris Tokyo Hong Kong

Prof. Dr. David T. Kelly
Hallstrom Institute of Cardiology, Royal Prince Alfred Hospital,
University of Sydney, Camperdown, N.S.W. 2050, Australia

ISBN-13: 978-3-540-51388-9 e-ISBN-13: 978-3-642-74911-7
DOI: 10.1007/978-3-642-74911-7

Library of Congress Cataloging-in-Publication Data
Asian Pacific Adalat Symposium (3rd : 1987 : Jakarta, Indonesia) 3rd Asian Pacific Adalat Symposium / David T. Kelly (Ed.). Includes index.
1. Nifedipine-Congresses. 2. Heart-Diseases-Chemotherapy-Congresses.
I. Kelly, David T. II. Title. III. Title: Third Asian Pacific Adalat Symposium.
RM666.N53A85 1987 616.1'061-dc20

Typesetting and printing: Zechnersche Buchdruckerei, Speyer
Bookbinding: J. Schäffer, Grünstadt

2127/3140-543210 - Printed on acid-free paper

Preface

These are the proceedings of the third Asian Pacific Adalat Symposium. The first was held in Tokyo in 1982 and the second in Sydney in 1985. We were honoured that the late Dr. Sukaman and his colleagues were able to host this third symposium in Jakarta.

This meeting was designed to contribute to and to promote international collaboration in cardiovascular research, and to help promote further knowledge and understanding about the treatment of vascular disease in the Asian Pacific area.

Nifedipine was originally investigated in the mid-1960s by Prof. Fleckenstein. His first results showed this drug was a powerful calcium antagonist which altered excitation contraction. At this time, there was a rapid development of knowledge about the pathophysiology of ischaemic heart disease, and thus the important pharmacological work on calcium antagonists such as nifedipine paralleled and complimented the newer understanding of coronary physiology in man. In a short time most therapy was designed to reduce myocardial oxygen consumption and demand. Coronary spasm was not thought to cause angina. When nifedipine was available for clinical investigation in 1968, it proved to be effective in patients with angina at rest. The clinical importance of spasm was later delineated and nifedipine became an effective treatment for ischaemic heart disease, numerous studies in the 1970s attesting to this, both for stable and unstable angina. Nifedipine also proved to be very effective in the treatment of hypertension and although used by several investigators in the 1970s, it was not officially approved for the treatment of hypertension until 1980. It is now one of the major drugs used worldwide for the treatment of hypertension and its use has increased since the long-acting or retard preparation was introduced. With the successful treatment of hypertension in contemporary society, many now develop and suffer from coronary artery disease, and a calcium antagonist such as nifedipine combines pharmacological properties that are ideal to treat this combined disorder and is also effective in the elderly.

The third Asian Pacific Adalat Symposium was divided into several sections.

The first on ischaemic heart disease highlighted the clinical effectiveness of the retard preparation of Adalat in stable angina. The use of Adalat in unstable angina was reviewed, as was its favourable effect on reperfusion following infarction. In addition nifedipine was shown to improve the abnormal relaxation of the left ventricle during ischaemia. The second section was on atherosclerosis, detailing the effects nifedipine may have on the development and progress of atherosclerosis both in cellular and animal experiments und also in humans. The third section was on hypertension, again showing the effectiveness of the retard preparation, how Adalat as monotherapy can effectively control hypertension long term. The final section discussed the effects of nifedipine on serum lipid metabolism and the all important effects on the coronary vascular circulation.

At its conclusion, the meeting was summarized by the late Dr. Sukaman. It is sad to note that this was one of his last official functions before his untimely death and I would like to acknowledge his many contributions to cardiology, especially in the Asian Pacific region. All participants wish to thank our Indonesian hosts and Bayer AG for such a stimulating meeting.

The incidence of both hypertension and coronary artery disease is increasing dramatically in Asian countries, in part due to the higher standards of living and increased life expectancy. It was appropriate that this third Asian Pacific Adalat symposium was held in Jakarta. The meeting was graciously opened by the Minister of Health for the Republic of Indonesian, the Honourable Dr. Suwardjono Surjaniograt, and in his excellent address he stressed the economic importance to the overall health system of the impressive rise in vascular mortality in the last decade in the Republic of Indonesia, emphasizing the government's interest in the diagnosis and successful treatment of vascular disease.

Sydney, Australia *D. T. Kelly*

Contents

Ischemic Heart Disease

Atherosclerosis

Contributors

Abarquez, R. F.
Philippine Heart Center, Medical Arts Building, East Avenue, Quezon City 1630, Philippines

Abdurahman, N.
Department of Internal Medicine, University of Indonesia, Dr. Cipto Mangunkusumo Hospital, Jakarta 11150, Indonesia

Abe, K.
Second Department of Internal Medicine, Tohoku University School of Medicine, 1-1, Seiryo-cho, Sendai 980, Japan

Abelardo, N. S.
Philippine Heart Center, Medical Arts Building, East Avenue, Quezon City 1630, Philippines

Arakawa, K.
Department of Internal Medicine, Fukuoka University Hospital, 7-45-1, Nanakuma, Jonan-ku, Fukuoka 814-01, Japan

Castillo, R. R.
Philippine Heart Center, Medical Arts Building, East Avenue, Quezon City 1630, Philippines

Enoveso, O. E.
Philippine Heart Center, Medical Arts Building, East Avenue, Quezon City 1630, Philippines

Fukuzaki, H.
First Department of Internal Medicine, Kobe University School of Medicine, 7-5-1 Kusunoki-cho, Chuo-ku, Kobe 650, Japan

Hirosumi, J.
Department of Geriatrics, Faculty of Medicine, University of Tokyo, 7-3-1 Hongo, Bunkyo-ku, Tokyo 113, Japan

Hirota, Y.
Department of Internal Medicine, Osaka Medical College, 2-7 Daigaku-cho, Takatsuki, Osaka 569, Japan

Hiwatari, M.
Second Department of Internal Medicine, Tohoku University School of Medicine, 1-1, Seiryo-cho, Sendai 980, Japan

Hugenholtz, P. G.
Erasmus Universiteit Rotterdam, Faculteit der Geneeskunde, Postbus 1738, 3000 DR Rotterdam, The Netherlands

Iimura, O.
Second Department of Internal Medicine, Sapporo Medical College, S-1, W-16, Chuo-ku, Sapporo 060, Japan

Ishikawa, Y.
First Department of Internal Medicine, Kobe University School of Medicine, 7-5-1 Kusunoki-cho, Chuo-ku, Kobe 650, Japan

Ismail, D.
Department of Internal Medicine, University of Indonesia, Dr. Cipto Mangunkusumo Hospital, Jakarta 11150, Indonesia

Jara, R. D.
Philippine Heart Center, Medical Arts Building, East Avenue, Quezon City 1630, Philippines

Kaku, K.
Department of Internal Medicine, Osaka Medical College, 2-7 Daigaku-cho, Takatsuki, Osaka 569, Japan

Kawai, C.
Third Department of Internal Medicine, Faculty of Medicine, Kyoto University, 54 Kawara-cho Shogoin, Sakyo-ku, Kyoto 606, Japan

Kawamura, K.
Department of Internal Medicine, Osaka Medical College, 2-7 Daigaku-cho, Takatsuki, Osaka 569, Japan

Kihara, Y.
Third Department of Internal Medicine, Faculty of Medicine, Kyoto University, 54 Kawara-cho Shogoin, Sakyo-ku, Kyoto 606, Japan

Kikuchi, K.
Second Department of Internal Medicine, Sapporo Medical College, S-1, W-16, Chuo-ku, Sapporo 060, Japan

Kita, Y.
Department of Internal Medicine, Osaka Medical College, 2-7 Daigaku-cho, Takatsuki, Osaka 569, Japan

Konishi, T.
Third Department of Internal Medicine, Faculty of Medicine, Kyoto University, 54 Kawara-cho Shogoin, Sakyo-ku, Kyoto 606, Japan

Kusunoki, J.
Department of Geriatrics, Faculty of Medicine, University of Tokyo, 7-3-1 Hongo, Bunkyo-ku, Tokyo 113, Japan

Mansjoer, H.
Department of Internal Medicine, University of Indonesia, Dr. Cipto Mangunkusumo Hospital, Jakarta 11150, Indonesia

Miyashita, H.
Second Department of Medicine, Teikyo University School of Medicine, 2-11-1 Kaga, Itabashi-ku, Tokyo 173, Japan

Miyazaki, Nobuhiro
First Department of Internal Medicine, Kobe University School of Medicine, 7-5-1 Kusunoki-cho, Chuo-ku, Kobe 650, Japan

Miyazaki, Shunichi
Third Department of Internal Medicine, Faculty of Medicine, Kyoto University, 54 Kawara-cho Shogoin, Sakyo-ku, Kyoto 606, Japan

Nakamura, Yasuyuki
Third Department of Internal Medicine, Faculty of Medicine, Kyoto University, 54 Kawara-cho Shogoin, Sakyo-ku, Kyoto 606, Japan

Nakamura, Yoshiro
Department of Medicine, Keio University School of Medicine, 35 Shinano-machi, Shinjuku-ku, Tokyo 160, Japan

Nonogi, H.
Third Department of Internal Medicine, Faculty of Medicine, Kyoto University, 54 Kawara-cho Shogoin, Sakyo-ku, Kyoto 606, Japan

Orimo, H.
Department of Geriatrics, Faculty of Medicine, University of Tokyo, 7-3-1 Hongo, Bunkyo-ku, Tokyo 113, Japan

Ouchi, Y.
Department of Geriatrics, Faculty of Medicine, University of Tokyo, 7-3-1 Hongo, Bunkyo-ku, Tokyo 113, Japan

Pun, C. O.
Department of Medicine, The Chinese University of Hong Kong, Prince of Wales Hospital, Shatin, NT, Hong Kong

Rahman, A. M.
Department of Internal Medicine, University of Indonesia, Dr. Cipto Mangunkusumo Hospital, Jakarta 11150, Indonesia

Saito, Takaharu
Department of Internal Medicine, Osaka Medical College, 2-7 Daigaku-cho, Takatsuki, Osaka 569, Japan

Saito, Tsuyoshi
Miyagi National Hospital, 100 Aza-Kassenhara, Takase, Yamamoto-cho, Watari-gun, Miyagi 989-22, Japan

Santoso, T.
Department of Internal Medicine, University of Indonesia, Dr. Cipto Mangunkusumo Hospital, Jakarta 11150, Indonesia

Sasaki, J.
Department of Internal Medicine, Fukuoka University Hospital, 7-45-1, Nanakuma, Jonan-ku, Fukuoka 814-01, Japan

Sasayama, S.
Second Department of Internal Medicine, Toyama Medical and Pharmaceutical University, 2630 Sugitani, Toyama 930-01, Japan

Sasou, S.
Miyagi National Hospital, 100 Aza-Kassenhara, Takase, Yamamoto-cho, Watari-gun, Miyagi 989-22, Japan

Shimamoto, K.
Second Department of Internal Medicine, Sapporo Medical College, S-1, W-16, Chuo-ku, Sapporo 060, Japan

Shimizu, G.
Department of Internal Medicine, Osaka Medical College,
2-7 Daigaku-cho, Takatsuki, Osaka 569, Japan

Sison, V. M.
Philippine Heart Center, Medical Arts Building, East Avenue,
Quezon City 1630, Philippines

Sugiarti, T.
Department of Internal Medicine, University of Indonesia,
Dr. Cipto Mangunkusumo Hospital, Jakarta 11150, Indonesia

Sugimoto, T.
Second Department of Medicine, Toyama Medical and
Pharmaceutical University, 2630 Sugitani, Toyama 930-01,
Japan

Sy, R. G.
Philippine Heart Center, Medical Arts Building, East Avenue,
Quezon City 1630, Philippines

Taniguchi, T.
First Department of Internal Medicine, Kobe University School
of Medicine, 7-5-1 Kusunoki-cho, Chuo-ku, Kobe 650, Japan

Toyama, Y.
Department of Cardiology, The Center for Adult Diseases,
1-3-3 Nakamichi, Higashinari-ku, Osaka 537, Japan

Ueda, K.
Department of Internal Medicine, Metropolitan Geriatric
Center, 35-2 Sakae-cho, Itabashi-ku, Tokyo, Japan

Vallance-Owen, J.
Department of Medicine, The Chinese University of Hong
Kong, Prince of Wales Hospital, Shatin, NT, Hong Kong

Wangge, M. N. T.
Department of Internal Medicine, University of Indonesia,
Dr. Cipto Mangunkusumo Hospital, Jakarta 11150, Indonesia

Watanabe, Masae
Department of Geriatrics, Faculty of Medicine, University
of Tokyo, 7-3-1 Hongo, Bunkyo-ku, Tokyo 113, Japan

Watanabe, Naoya
First Department of Internal Medicine, Kobe University School of Medicine, 7-5-1 Kusunoki-cho, Chuo-ku, Kobe 650, Japan

Watanabe, Yoshio
Institute for Experimental Animal, Kobe University School of Medicine, 7-5-1 Kusunoki-cho, Chuo-ku, Kobe 650, Japan

Woo, K. S.
Department of Medicine, The Chinese University of Hong Kong, Prince of Wales Hospital, Shatin, NT, Hong Kong

Yabe, Y.
Cardiovascular Diagnostic Laboratory Center, Toho University School of Medicine, 6-11-1 Omori-Nishi, Ota-ku, Tokyo 143, Japan

Yoshinaga, K.
Second Department of Internal Medicine, Tohoku University School of Medicine, 1-1, Seiryo-cho, Sendai 980, Japan

Ischemic Heart Disease

Study on the Clinical Effectiveness of Adalat L Tablet for Angina Pectoris: A Double-blind Study with Adalat as a Reference Drug

Y. Nakamura[1], H. Miyashita[2], O. Iimura[3], K. Ueda[4], T. Sugimoto[5], and Y. Toyama[6]

Introduction

Nifedipine is a potent Ca^{2+} antagonist and is effective not only for vasospastic angina but also for stable-effort angina [1]. Nifedipine was initially supplied as a liquid-filled capsule formulation with rapid- but short-acting characteristics. The nifedipine capsule is generally administered every 8 h, however the administration of nifedipine t.i.d. cannot control episodes of the variant form of angina pectoris which occur early in the morning [2]. Adalat L (Bayer) was therefore developed for the purpose of producing a long-acting effect. It has been reported that 12 h after oral administration of 20 mg Adalat L, its plasma concentration was still higher than the minimal effective level [3].

In our previous open study [4], 20 mg oral Adalat L b.i.d. was revealed to have a very good effect in controlling both vasospastic and stable-effort angina. Here we have tried to advance our studies to the next phase of the clinical trial of Adalat L. The purpose of this study was to compare the antianginal effect of 20 mg Adalat L b.i.d. with that of 10 mg nifedipine t.i.d. by means of a double-blind multicenter study.

Methods

Subjects: Patients with rest and/or effort angina pectoris were selected for this study according to the following criteria. The frequency of angina episodes which could be controlled by sublingual nitroglycerin or isosorbide dinitrate was specified to be at least three per week but not more than five per

[1] Department of Medicine, Keio University School of Medicine
[2] Second Department of Medicine, Teikyo University School of Medicine
[3] Second Department of Medicine, Sapporo Medical College
[4] Department of Internal Medicine, Tokyo Metropolitan Geriatric Hospital
[5] Second Department of Medicine, Toyama Medical and Pharmaceutical University Faculty of Medicine
[6] Department of Cardiology, The Center for Adult Diseases, Osaka, Japan

day, with minimal day-to-day or week-to-week variation. In addition, it was necessary for the electrocardiogram of these patients to have revealed ischemic ST-T change at rest and/or during anginal attack or exercise. The age of patients was between 40 and 75 years. Informed consent was obtained from each patient.

The following patients were excluded from this study:

(a) those with congestive heart failure, uncontrolled hypertension, hyper- or hypo- thyroidism, severe anemia, valvular heart disease, atrioventricular block, or insulin-dependent diabetes mellitus;
(b) those with acute myocardial infarction within 6 months from onset;
(c) those with severe dysfunction of the liver or kidney;
(d) those pregnant or possibly pregnant;
(e) those who for various reasons were considered to be unsuitable for the study.

Both in- and outpatients were included in this study, but outpatients who were hospitalized or inpatients who were discharged during this study were excluded from the analysis.

Study Design and Assessment: All patients were observed during a 2-week period on placebo (placebo period) to ensure they were in a stable clinical stage. The use of β-blockers or calcium antagonists other than the drugs used in this study and so-called coronary vasodilators was prohibited throughout this study. Sedatives, diuretics, and antihypertensives which had previously been administered chronically were continued without change in their doses during the study period. From the 3rd week (active period), patients were randomized, and 20 mg Adalat L b.i.d. with a placebo of nifedipine t.i.d. or 10 mg nifedipine t.i.d. with a placebo of Adalat L b.i.d. was given on a double-blind basis for 4 weeks.

Subjective symptoms including the frequency, character, intensity and precipitation of angina, nitroglycerin consumption, work capacity, and impression of drug effects were reported by means of a patient diary. Patients' reports were assessed by investigators, and subjective improvement was classified as markedly improved, improved, slightly improved, unchanged, or deteriorated. Chest X-ray film, electrocardiogram at rest and after exercise by the double Master's two-step test or treadmill test, and blood and urine samples for laboratory examinations, were taken during the placebo period and at the end of the active period. Blood pressure and heart rate were measured every 2 weeks. Evaluations of electrocardiogram at rest and after exercise were done according to the criteria shown in Figs. 1 and 2.

The medical criteria for withdrawal from the study were intercurrent procedures that might influence the evaluation of the effects of the two drugs administered in this study. When mild complications considered to be caused by the Ca^{2+} antagonists were suspected, the patient was carefully observed without change in the dosage of the drugs, but when the degree of complication

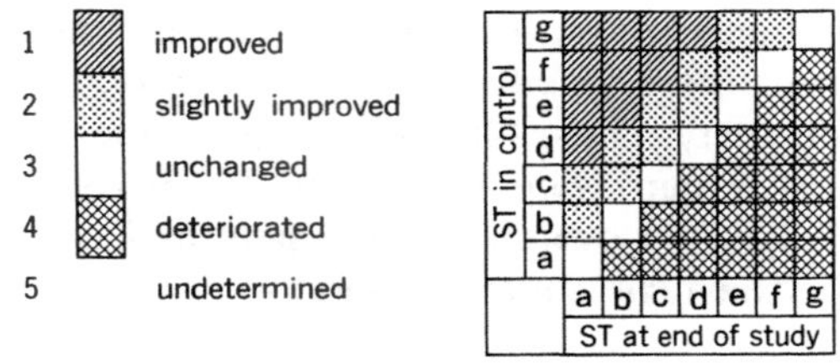

a normal
b ST depression ≥ 1 mm J type
c ST depression < 0.5 mm Horizontal
d ST depression < 0.5 mm Downsloping
e ST depression ≥ 0.5 mm (<1mm) ischemic
f ST depression ≥ 1 mm ischemic
g ST depression ≥ 2 mm ischemic

Fig. 1. Evaluation of ECG changes at rest

	ST depression by exercise at end of study − ST depression by exercise in control (ΔST)
1. improved	∼ −1.0 mm
2. slightly improved	−0.9 ∼ −0.5
3. unchanged	−0.4 ∼ +0.4
4. deteriorated	+0.4 ∼
5. undetermined	

Fig. 2. Evaluation of ECG changes during exercise

was moderate or severe, the drugs were eliminated and treatment for the complication was performed if it was necessary.

Overall improvement was evaluated from subjective improvement and ECG changes according to five grades. Safety was assessed from the view point of side and adverse effects, in consideration of any changes in laboratory data, according to four grades. Usefulness was evaluated in terms of overall improvement and safety according to five grades, by comparing data obtained at onset to those at the end of the study.

Statistics: The Mann-Whitney *U* test or Sign test was used for nonparametric statistics, e.g., the comparison of subjective improvement between nifedipine and Adalat L groups. The χ^2 test was used for parametric statistics. Values for p of less than 0.05 were considered to be significant.

Results

Study Groups and Degree of Similarity in Their Background: Of the 118 patients who were randomly assigned, 57 received Adalat L and 61 nifedipine, but four were excluded because of failure to follow the study protocol. Nine patients whose frequency of angina episodes in the placebo period did not meet those specified in the study protocol were subjected only to evaluation of safety. Thus, 105 patients (51 in the Adalat L group and 54 in the nifedipine group) were included in the analysis of group comparison of subjective, ECG, and overall improvement and usefulness. There were no differences between clinical and laboratory variables in the two groups.

Withdrawal from the Study: Of eight patients (five in the Adalat L group and three in the nifedipine group) withdrawn from the study, two in the Adalat L group revealed subjective deterioration. In the other six patients, medication was discontinued because of side effects of the test drugs. Subjective, ECG, and overall improvement were evaluated at the end of the 2nd week of the active period, if data were available, in all but one who was included in only the safety analysis.

Subjective Improvement: Basic data used for the evaluation of subjective improvement are presented in Figs. 3–5. An increase in the frequency of anginal attack associated with an increase in the consumption of nitrate in the Adalat L group was seen in the 3rd week of the active period. Improvement of work capacity as reflected in patients' impressions was more marked in the Adalat L group in the 1st week of the active period in comparison with the nifedipine group. These minimal differences did not affect the assessment of subjective improvement, which was done by comparing the improvement from the end of the placebo period to the end of the active period (Table 1). The percent-

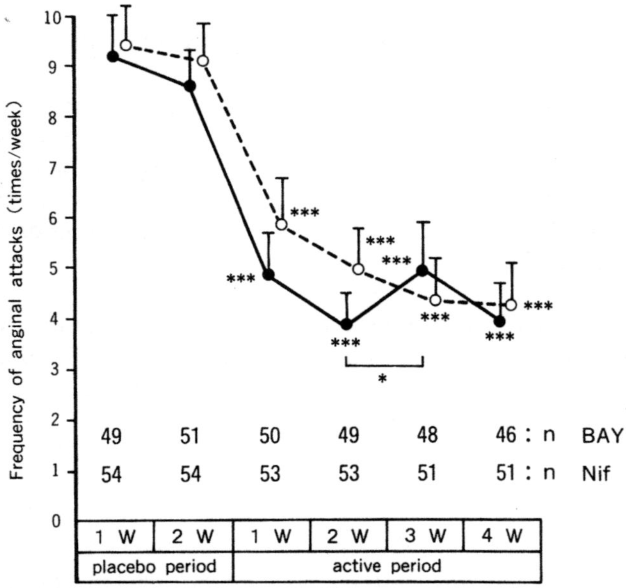

Fig. 3. Frequency of anginal attacks per week. *Solid line,* Adalat L (*BAY*); *broken line,* nifedipine (*Nif*); * $p<0.05$; *** $p<0.001$ (in comparison to placebo in 2nd week)

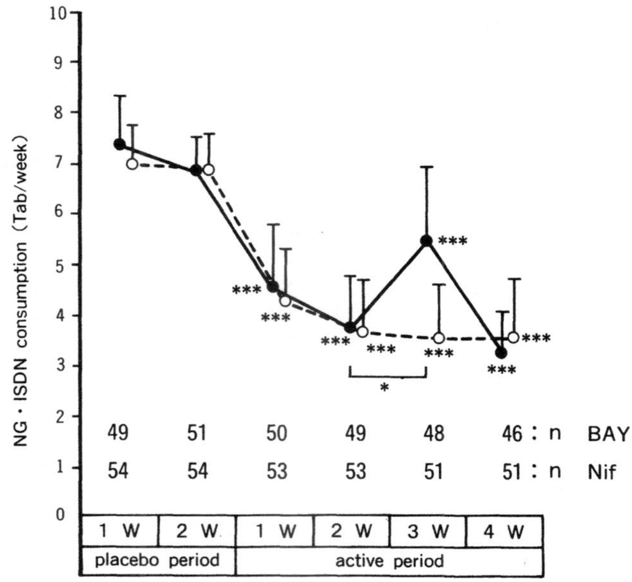

Fig. 4. Consumption of nitroglycerin (*NG*) or isosorbide dinitrate (*ISDN*) per week. *Solid line,* Adalat L (*BAY*); *broken line,* nifedipine (*Nif*); * $p<0.05$; *** $p<0.001$ (in comparison to placebo in 2nd week)

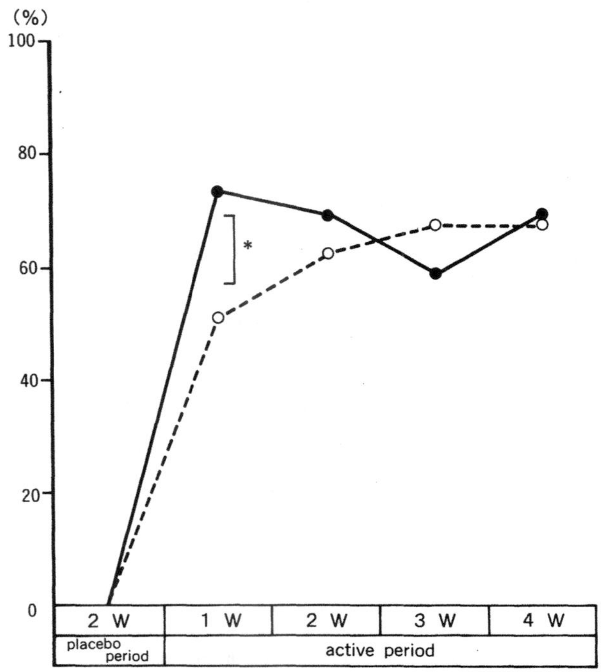

Fig. 5. Patients' impressions of improvement per week. Percentage of patients who were improved subjectively in comparison to the previous week. *Solid line,* Adalat L ($n=50$); *broken line,* nifedipine ($n=54$); * $p<0.05$

age of markedly improved cases in the nifedipine group was significantly higher than that in the Adalat L group.

ECG Changes: Exercise ECG was improved or slightly improved by the test drugs in 54%–56% of the patients, but no difference was seen between ECG changes at rest and after exercise in the Adalat L and nifedipine groups (Tables 2, 3).

Table 1. Assessment of subjective improvement

	Markedly improved	Improved	Slightly improved	Unchanged	Deteriorated	Total	Unknown
Adalat L	8 (15.7)	29 (56.9)	8 (15.7)	4 (7.8)	2 (3.9)	51 (100.0)	0
	37 (72.5)						
Nifedipine	19 (35.8)	16 (30.2)	8 (15.1)	10 (18.9)	0 (0)	53 (100.0)	1
	35 (66.0)						

U test, NS; χ^2 test, significant difference ($p<0.05$) in "markedly improved". Percentages in parentheses.

Table 2. Assessment of ECG improvement at rest

	Improved	Slightly improved	Unchanged	Deteriorated	Total	Undetermined
Adalat L	3 (6.3)	8 (16.7)	34 (70.8)	3 (6.3)	48 (100.0)	3
	11 (22.9)					
Nifedipine	5 (10.0)	7 (14.0)	37 (74.0)	1 (2.0)	50 (100.0)	4
	12 (24.0)					

U and χ^2 tests, NS. Percentages in parentheses.

Table 3. Assessment of exercise ECG improvement

	Improved	Slightly improved	Unchanged	Deteriorated	Total	Undetermined
Adalat L	10 (27.0)	10 (27.0)	17 (45.9)	0 (0)	37 (100.0)	14
	20 (54.1)					
Nifedipine	12 (29.3)	11 (26.8)	17 (41.5)	1 (2.4)	41 (100.0)	13
	23 (56.1)					

U and χ^2 tests, NS. Percentages in parentheses.

Overall Improvement: There was no difference between the degree of overall improvement in the two groups (Table 4).

Safety: Acute myocardial infarction occurred in one patient in the Adalat L group, but it could not be determined whether this was due to the drug or not. Side effects occurred in 8.8% of Adalat L cases and in 17.5% of nifedipine cases. This difference was not statistically significant. Of 15 patients who showed side effects, 10 complained of symptoms related to vasodilation. Other side effects were gastrointestinal disturbances. Assessment of safety is shown in Table 5. There was no difference between the levels of safety assessed in the two groups.

Usefulness: There was no difference in the degree of usefulness evaluated in the two groups (Table 6).

Table 4. Assessment of overall improvement

	Markedly improved	Improved	Slightly improved	Unchanged	Deteriorated	Total	Unknown
Adalat L	8 (15.7)	29 (56.9)	7 (13.7)	5 (9.8)	2 (3.9)	51 (100.0)	0
	37 (72.5)						
Nifedipine	11 (20.8)	25 (47.2)	9 (17.0)	8 (15.1)	0 (0)	53 (100.0)	1
	36 (67.9)						

U and χ^2 tests, NS. Percentages in parentheses.

Table 5. Assessment of safety

	No side effects	Mild side effects, study continued	Moderate side effects, study discontinued but no treatment necessary	Severe side effects, study discontinued and treatment necessary	Total
Adalat L	52 (91.2)	2 (3.5)	3 (5.3)	0 (0)	57 (100.0)
		5 (8.8)			
Nifedipine	47 (82.5)	7 (12.3)	2 (3.5)	1 (1.8)	57 (100.0)
		10 (17.5)			

U and χ^2 tests, NS. Percentages in parentheses.

Table 6. Assessment of usefulness

	Very useful	Useful	Slightly useful	Not useful	Prohibited from use	Total	Unknown
Adalat L	10 (19.6)	27 (52.9)	9 (17.6)	4 (7.8)	1 (2.0)	51 (100.0)	0
	37 (72.5)						
Nifedipine	13 (24.1)	24 (44.4)	10 (18.5)	6 (11.1)	1 (1.9)	54 (100.0)	0
	37 (68.5)						

U and χ^2 tests, NS. Percentages in parentheses.

Discussion

The Protocol: This protocol, in which not only patients with effort angina but also those with rest angina were included, leads to the question as to whether the effect of the treatment of vasospastic angina may be evaluated by the same method as that for fixed coronary restriction angina. An objection may be raised to the assessment of the antianginal effect of the drugs from the viewpoint of reduction in the frequency of anginal episodes in cases of effort angina due to the lack of objective findings, even though the stability of occurrence of anginal episodes was confirmed when the patients were entered into this study. At the same time, the evaluation of antianginal effect by changes in exercise tolerance in patients with rest angina may also be questioned. The many reported cases of coronary spasm with ST depression upon anginal attack and during exercise [5–8] have confused the clinical concept of vasospastic angina. In this study, although the relative distribution of patients with vasospastic angina in the respective groups was not known, there was no statistically significant difference in the background detected between the patients treated with nifedipine and those treated with Adalat L. At present, strict exclusion of cases of vasospastic angina from those of effort angina is impossible. The four cases of rest or variant angina included in each group in this study might not affect the results. In spite of these limitations in the protocol employed, comparison of the antianginal effect of different formulations but the same ingredient of nifedipine was considered to be reasonable in this study.

Subjective Improvement: Subjectively, more markedly improved cases were seen in the nifedipine group than in the Adalat L group, while reduction in the frequency of anginal episodes was slightly more marked in the Adalat L group than in the nifedipine group. Thus, subjective improvement may not be seen simply as a reflection of a decrease in the frequency of anginal episodes. Although several factors are likely to have affected this assessment, analysis of these factors was unable to provide any conclusions in this study.

Electrocardiographic Changes: Coronary vasodilators would not be expected to improve ECG findings at rest in patients with stable chronic ischemic heart disease, although exercise ECG should be improved [9]. In this study, exercise testing was performed by the double Master's two-step test in almost all cases, and no increase in work capacity by the drugs could be shown. The magnitude of ST segment depression is believed to indicate the degree of ischemia. It has been reported that the incidence of future coronary events within 6 years is greater in patients with an increased magnitude of ST depression after exercise approximately equivalent to that of a single Master's test [10]. The improvement in the magnitude of ST depression after the double Master's test seen in about 55% of the patients in both the nifedipine and Adalat L groups could thus be recorded as evidence of the effect of the drugs.

References

1. Kimura E, Mabuchi G, Kikuchi H (1973) Clinical evaluation of effect of nifedipine on angina pectoris by sequential analysis. In: Hashimoto K, Kimura E, Kobayashi T (eds) Proceedings of first international nifedipine symposium, Tokyo, 1973. University of Tokyo Press, Tokyo, p 155
2. Muller JE, Gunter SJ (1978) Nifedipine therapy for Prinzmetal's angina. Circulation 57:137
3. Hata T, Shigematsu H, Tsushima M et al. (1982) On the blood concentration and safety of nifedipine tablet in the healthy people (in Japanese). Rinsho To Kenkyu 59:1699
4. Iimura S, Miyashita H, Nakamura Y et al. (1982) Prevention of anginal attack by BAY a 1040; a pilot study (in Japanese). Rinsho To Kenkyu 59:3053
5. Specchia G, DeServi S, Falcone C et al. (1979) Coronary arterial spasm as a cause of exercise-induced ST segment elevation in patients with variant angina. Circulation 59:948
6. Yasue H, Omote S, Takizawa A et al. (1979) Exertional angina pectoris caused by coronary artery spasm: effects of various drugs. Am J Cardiol 43:647
7. Maseri A, Servi S, DeNes M et al. (1978) Variant angina: one aspect of a continuous spectrum of vasospastic myocardial ischemia. Am J Cardiol 42:1019
8. Yasue H, Omote S, Takizawa A et al. (1981) Comparison of coronary arteriographic findings during angina pectoris associated with ST segment elevation or depression. Am J Cardiol 47:539
9. Amsterdam EA, Price JE, Berman D et al. (1977) Exercise testing in the indirect assessment of myocardial oxygen consumption: application for evaluation of mechanism and therapy of angina pectoris. In: Amsterdam EA, Wilmore JH, DeMaria AM (eds) Exercise in cardiovascular health and disease. Yorke, New York, p 218
10. Ellestad MH, Allen WH, Stuart RJ (1978) Diagnostic and prognostic information derived from exercise testing. In: Wenger NK (ed) Exercise and the heart. Cardiovasc Clin 9 (3): 33

Nifedipine-Induced Reperfusion in Stable Angina and Postinfarction Cases

R. F. Abarquez[1], V. M. Sison[1], R. G. Sy[1], N. S. Abelardo[1], R. R. Castillo[1], R. D. Jara[1], and O. E. Enoveso[1]

Introduction

Most of the diagnostic and therapeutic approaches to angina pectoris focus on epicardial coronary artery abnormalities. Yet, pathophysiologic and clinical manifestations are not always related to the degree or extent of the coronary pathology. Although significant occlusive disease with total coronary flow reduction results in transmural pathology, patients may have no angina, ischemia, electrophysiologic changes, or lactate production at rest [1–4], some may have angina due to subendocardial ischemia [5–6], and 28%–50% may have no myocardial infarction [7–9]. After coronary bypass surgery of noninfarction cases only 21%–75% have improved wall motion [10–12]. Thus, survival is predicted by the degree of residual left ventricular dysfunction rather than by the number or extent of diseased vessels [13]. Likewise, factors other than fixed obstuctive lesions of the epicardial vessels may contribute to ventricular function.

Patients with classical angina with significant ST-segment depression during an exercise test plus the presence of exercise-induced hypoperfusion on thallium scintigraphy usually merit coronary arteriography to exclude surgically remediable epicardial fixed obstructive disease. After an infarct, left-main or triple-vessel disease may be excluded if thallium imaging is negative outside the infarct zone since exercise-induced ST-segment depressions with perfusion defect usually reflect advanced coronary artery disease [14–19]. However, exercise-induced ST-segment depression as well as postinfarction angina may be related to vasospastic mechanisms [20]. The objective of this study, therefore, is to determine whether calcium blockers can reverse or lead to improvement in stress-induced ischemia in patients with implied fixed obstructive coronary artery disease.

[1] Philippine Heart Center, Medical Arts Building, Quezon City, Philippines

Methods

Nineteen patients with stable angina of effort for at least 1 month and five postinfarction patients had treadmill tests showing ST-segment changes of at least 0.1 mV. None had clinically associated significant illness. No one was on digitalis or on antiarrhythmic or psychotrophic agents. Bundle branch block and other conduction abnormalities were not present in the resting ECG.

All patients gave written informed consent on entry into the study and before each exercise testing session. Exercise was terminated if there were symptoms such as effort-induced chest pain, dyspnea, fatiguability, leg cramps, or dizziness; if there was a decrease in systolic pressure of at least 10 mmHg below the peak value obtained at the previous stage of exercise; or if ventricular (at least three successive) premature beats occurred. At peak exercise 1.5 mCi thallium 201 (T-201) was injected intravenously, and exercise was continued for an additional 60s. Perfusion imaging was obtained using an Ohio Nuclear series with 150 Interphase and an ADAC computer System I. Twelve lead ECG and blood pressure measurements were recorded at rest, before exercise testing, at the end of each 3-min stage of exercise, and 1, 2, 3, 5, and 8 min after exercise. During the recovery period, myocardial imaging was recorded using a scintillation camera set for 140 KeV with a low-energy all-purpose parallel volt collimator. Data collection was begun in all cases within 10 min of radioactive tracer injection. Data was collected in each of the three projections – anterior, left anterior oblique at 30°, and left lateral view. Between 250000 and 300000 counts were collected per projection. All images were reproduced using a Polaroid photograph obtained directly from the camera cathode-ray display. In addition, the data was collected and viewed on an ADAC Computer Medical Data System I. Imaging and data collections were repeated 4 h after exercise to assess redistribution of the isotope.

Exercise and postexercise electrocardiograms were analyzed for positive or negative response. A positive response was defined as either a horizontal or down-sloping ST-segment depression of 1 mm 0.08 s after the J-point or a 1-mm ST-segment elevation. Thallium 201 images were independently assessed semiquantitatively by interpreters unaware of the patient's history and electrocardiographic exercise test results. The borders of hypoperfused area were identified in each view and with a center point; the angles subtending the hypoperfused area were computed and recorded. After the exercise test and thallium scintigraphy, nifedipine 10 mg three times per day for 1 week was initially started in order to avoid side effects and associated tachycardia. Subsequently, the dose was increased to 20 mg three times per day in some patients for a period of at least 1 month. After this time a repeat treadmill test with T-201 imaging as in the pretreatment period was performed. Coronary arteriography was performed in six cases with ergonovine injection test in one case done in a center in the United States. The parameters for comparison before and after nifedipine were the symptom-limited exercise capacity or treadmill duration in minutes, ST-segment changes, heart rate, systolic blood pressure, and rate pressure product × 10^2. The angles subtending the exercise-induced T-201-hypoperfused areas on anterior, left anterior oblique, and lateral views were determined. Student's *T* test and Wilcoxon's *U* test were used for analysis. A *p* value of less than .05 was accepted as statistically significant.

Results

Table 1 presents the initial profile of the 24 patients. Patients 1–7 had treadmill test while patients 8–24 had treadmill test and T-201 imaging before and after nifedipine, and patients 11, 13, 15, 17, 18, 23, and 24 had T-201 imaging only after oral nifedipine. Patients 9, 17, 18, 19, 22, and 24 had coronary arteriography performed in various medical centers in the United States showing insignificant (less than 50%) occlusive disease. Patient number 24 also had a positive ergonovine test before oral nifedipine. There were 8 women and 16 men; ages ranged from 29 to 66 years (mean, 50 ± 11 years). Angina duration was from 1 month to 11 years (mean, 3.2 years). The respective risk profiles are shown in Table 1; the daily nifedipine dose given with associated medication administered in some cases is also shown. Case 24 received, however, verapamil 240 mg per day because of a tendency to tachycardia on nifedipine.

Table 2 shows that maximal heart rate increased on nifedipine from 121.3 ± 25.3 to 137.2 ± 23.6 ($p<.01$) while the rate-pressure product increased from 202.5 ± 59.39 to 227 ± 57.5 ($p<.05$). Systolic blood pressure was not significantly different at end of exercise. At comparable load, after nifedipine systolic blood pressure was diminished from 167.9 ± 31.2 to 158 ± 22.53 ($p<.05$), and heart rate increased from 114.54 ± 21.8 to 122 ± 20.9 ($p<.05$) without significant changes in the rate-pressure product.

Table 3 shows that nifedipine reduced the level of ST-segment depression from −2.4 ± 0.95 mm to −0.83 ± 0.84 ($p<.001$). ST-segment elevation in three cases (numbers 8, 16, and 20) of 1.66 ± 0.28 after nifedipine dropped to 0 ($p<.001$). The treadmill duration measured after nifedipine increased from 9.74 ± 4.6 to 11.98 ± 4.1 min ($p<.05$). In all views the angle subtending the exercise-induced hypoperfused area was significantly reduced by nifedipine: from 91.3 ± 25.01° to 36.2 ± 44.94° on anterior view ($p<.01$), from 95.2 ± 27.67° to 39.7 ± 45.72° on left anterior oblique view ($p<.01$), and from 70.4 ± 41.12° to 22.9 ± 29.77° on left lateral view ($p<.01$), with a total reduction from 256.9 ± 77.6° to 99.8 ± 119° ($p<.001$). Of the 14 cases with exercise-induced thallium-hypoperfused area before nifedipine, 12 (70%) had normal thallium scintigraphy after nifedipine.

Table 4 and Fig. 1 show that ST-segment depressions are noted as early as stage 1 and persist until late in the recovery period. After nifedipine the degree of ST-segment drop reverted closer to ECG baseline levels. Subsequent follow-up of all cases showed improved functional capacity and total relief of angina.

Table 1. Initial patient profiles

Patient	Age (years)	Sex	Anginal duration	Risk profile	Medication/day
1. N.B.	63	M	3 years	Diabetes	Adalat 30 mg
2. J.C.	61	F	3 months	Hypertension, smoking	Adalat 30 mg
3. V.E.	33	F	1 year	None	Adalat 30 mg
4. A.E.	55	F	3 months	Hypercholesterolemia	Adalat 30 mg
5. L.C.	42	M	1 year	Hypertension, hypercholesterolemia	Adalat 30 mg
6. R.B.	48	F	1 year	Hypertension	Adalat 30 mg
7. B.D.	29	F	3 months	None	Adalat 30 mg
8. E.L.	38	M	1 month	None	Adalat 60 mg
9. L.M.[a]	58	M	5 years	None	Adalat 30 mg
10. E.U.	66	M	1.5 years	Diabetes, hyperuricemia, hypertension	Adalat 45 mg, diuretics
11. J.A.	55	M	2 years	None	Adalat 30 mg
12. D.T.	60	M	4 years	Diabetes, hypertension	Adalat 30 mg
13. V.R.	62	M	1 month	None	Adalat 30 mg
14. R.P.	48	M	8 years	Hyperuricemia	Adalat 60 mg, diuretics
15. F.Z.	58	F	10 years	Hypertension	Adalat 30 mg, diuretics
16. M.L.	45	M	10 months	Hypercholesterolemia, hyperuricemia	Adalat 30 mg
17. K.Y.S.[a]	56	M	6 years	Hyperuricemia	Adalat 30 mg, diuretics
18. R.C.[a]	35	M	3 years	Hypertension	Adalat 30 mg
19. G.L.[a]	45	F	3 months	Hypertension	Adalat 30 mg
20. J.C.	52	M	9 years	Diabetes, hypercholesterolemia	Adalat 15 mg
21. A.R.	41	M	1 month	Smoking, hypercholesterolemia	Adalat 45 mg
22. A.R.[a]	43	M	4 years	Hypertension	Adalat 30 mg
23. C.S.	66	M	11 years	None	Adalat 15 mg, diuretics
24. A.M.S.[b]	41	F	3 years	Borderline hypertension	Verapamil 240 mg

Patients 1–7 had treadmill test only. Patients 8–24 had treadmill test and thallium imaging – before and after nifedipine with numbers 11, 13, 15, 17, 18, 23, and 24 having thallium imaging only after nifedipine administration. Patients 9, 17, 18, 19, 22, and 24 had insufficient coronary arteriographic findings and 24 had a positive ergonovine test before nifedipine administration.

[a] Insignificant angiography.

[b] Angiography with positive ergonovine test.

Table 2. Blood pressure, heart rate, and rate-pressure product

Patient	Age (years)	Sex	Systolic blood pressure						Heart rate						Rate pressure product × 10^2					
			Resting		Comparable load		End of exercise		Resting		Comparable load		End of exercise		Resting		Comparable load		End of exercise	
			C	N	C	N	C	N	C	N	C	N	C	N	C	N	C	N	C	N
1. N.B.	63	M	130	117	180	167	160	156	50	75	83	98	83	121	65	87	149	162	132	188
2. J.C.	61	F	150	130	200	157	200	190	71	68	100	109	115	125	196	88	200	172	200	237
3. V.E.	33	F	100	120	130	128	130	120	71	83	103	109	103	136	71	99	133	151	103	163
4. A.E.	55	F	130	108	200	170	200	170	75	93	125	132	125	150	97	100	250	225	250	255
5. L.C.	42	F	100	100	180	170	180	160	68	107	125	153	150	168	68	107	225	265	227	268
6. R.B.	48	F	150	120	170	170	170	170	115	100	125	133	125	168	172	120	212	225	212	285
7. B.D.	29	F	100	100	140	120	140	130	93	107	136	156	150	168	93	107	190	187	210	218
8. E.L.	38	M	110	110	160	160	160	170	78	71	166	160	166	185	85	78	265	256	265	314
9. L.M.[a]	58	M	140	140	190	160	190	210	58	68	115	100	115	150	81	95	218	160	218	315
10. E.U.	66	M	160	140	240	200	240	200	58	120	120	125	120	125	93	81	288	250	288	250
11. J.A.	55	M	110	110	150	156	150	156	54	58	100	134	100	150	59	64	150	209	150	234
12. D.T.	60	M	130	140	170	140	180	140	62	55	100	100	107	100	81	77	170	140	192	140
13. V.R.	62	M	130	130	200	158	200	174	70	68	142	158	142	174	91	111	284	316	284	365
14. R.P.	48	M	140	130	140	170	130	170	60	71	100	115	120	115	84	92	140	196	156	196
15. F.Z.	58	M	100	140	170	170	170	180	68	92	88	115	88	125	88	129	150	196	150	225
16. M.L.	45	M	110	100	120	110	120	134	66	71	75	88	75	140	73	71	90	97	90	182
17. K.Y.S.[a]	56	M	120	114	160	170	160	180	65	71	136	115	136	140	96	81	200	196	200	252
18. R.C.[a]	35	M	120	150	190	170	190	170	75	55	136	107	136	107	90	182	258	182	258	182
19. G.L.[a]	45	M	120	120	120	120	120	120	58	71	83	107	83	110	70	85	100	128	100	132
20. J.C.	52	M	110	110	150	170	170	170	71	65	134	130	150	130	78	72	210	221	255	221
21. A.R.	41	M	110	100	150	160	200	160	78	68	107	115	125	115	86	68	161	184	250	184
22. A.R.[a]	43	M	130	140	170	160	170	160	68	62	107	107	107	107	88	87	182	171	182	171
23. C.S.	66	M	160	160	220	200	220	200	89	75	126	134	126	134	142	120	277	268	277	268
24. A.M.S.[b]	41	F	160	160	130	136	136	136	94	83	117	150	165	150	113	100	152	204	211	204
$n=$			24	24	24	24	24	24	24	24	24	24	24	24	24	24	24	24	24	24
$Q=$			18.63	17.05	31.20	22.53	31.59	24.38	14.63	15.32	21.8	20.9	25.3	23.6	24.5	23.64	56.69	49.95	59.39	57.50
$\bar{X}=$			124.16	122.9	167.9	158.0	170.2	163.6	71.45	75.54	114.5	122	121.3	137.2	90.46	137.2	193.6	194.4	202.5	227.04
$p=$			NS		<.05		NS		NS		<.05		<.01		NS		NS		<.05	

C, Control; N, nifedipine.
[a] Insignificant angiography.
[b] Angiography with positive ergonovine test.

Table 3. Post-myocardial infarction, ST-segment depression/elevation, and thallium 201 imaging

Patient	PMI	ST-segment depression/elevation		Treadmill duration (min)		Thallium 201 imaging views: Anterior		Left anterior oblique		Left lateral		Total	
		C	N	C	N	C	N	C	N	C	N	C	N
1. N.B.		−3.0	−2.5	12.0	12.0	None	None	None	None	None	None	None	None
2. J.C.		−2.5	−2.5	8.0	12.0	None	None	None	None	None	None	None	None
3. V.E.		−3.0	−0.5	4.0	12.0	None	None	None	None	None	None	None	None
4. A.E.		−3.5	−0.5	12.0	14.0	None	None	None	None	None	None	None	None
5. L.C.		−2.0	−0.5	22.0	24.0	None	None	None	None	None	None	None	None
6. R.B.		−1.0	−1.0	6.0	14.0	None	None	None	None	None	None	None	None
7. B.D.		−1.0	−0.5	14.0	14.6	None	None	None	None	None	None	None	None
8. E.L.		1.5	0.0	12.0	15.0	100	0	65	0	85	0	250	0
9. L.M.		−2.0[b]	0.0	7.30	17.0	90	0	110	0	0	0	200	0
10. E.U.		−2.5	−1.5	10.35	12.30	83	0	75	0	90	0	248	0
11. J.A.		−5.0	−1.0	9.0	10.0	None	0	None	0	None	0	None	0
12. D.T.		−2.0	−1.0	8.0	8.0	105	72	90	80	65	55	260	207
13. V.R.		−2.5	0.0	12.0	18.0	None	0	None	0	None	0	None	0
14. R.P.	+	−2.5	−2.0	10.0	9.0	95	85	100	75	45	39	240	199
15. F.Z.		−1.0	0.0	6.0	7.5	None	0	None	0	None	0	None	0
16. M.L.	+	1.5	0.0	1.30	13.0	40	35	57	52	19	15	116	102
17. K.Y.S.		−2.5[b]	0.0	10.0	11.0	None	0	None	0	None	0	None	0
18. R.C.		−2.5[b]	−1.0	10.0	12.0	None	0	None	0	None	0	None	0
19. G.L.	+	−2.5[b]	−2.0	2.0	4.0	125	125	155	125	145	85	425	335
20. J.C.	+	2.0	0.0	16.0	12.0	60	0	110	0	80	0	250	0
21. A.R.		−1.5	0.0	15.0	11.0	105	0	100	0	95	0	300	0
22. A.R.	+	−1.5[b]	−1.0	8.0	7.0	110	45	90	65	80	35	280	145
23. C.S.		−3.0	0.0	6.0	9.0	None	0	None	0	None	0	None	0
24. A.M.S.		−3.5[c]	0.0	13.0	9.15	None	0	None	0	None	0	None	0
n=	3[a] 3	21	21	24	24	10	10	10	10	10	10	10	10
$\underline{Q}$=	0.28 0	0.95	0.84	4.60	4.10	25.01	44.94	27.67	45.72	41.12	29.77	77.60	119.00
$\bar{X}$=	1.66	−2.40	−0.83	9.74	11.98	91.30	36.20	95.20	39.70	70.40	22.90	256.90	98.80
p=	<.001	<.001		<.05		<.01		<.01		<.01		<.001	

PMI, Post-myocardial infarction; C, Control; N, nifedipine.
[a] ST elevation. [b] Insignificant angiography. [c] Angiography with positive ergonovine test.

Table 4. ST-segment depression (mm)

Patient	Age (years)	Sex	Stage 0		1		2		3		4		Time after exercise 2 min		5 min		8 min	
			C	N	C	N	C	N	C	N	C	N	C	N	C	N	C	N
1. N.B.	63	M																
2. J.C.	61	F																
3. V.E.	33	F																
4. A.E.	55	F																
5. L.C.	42	M																
6. R.B.	48	F																
7. B.D.	29	F																
8. F.L.	38	M																
9. L.M.[a]	58	M	0	0	0	0	0.5	0	1.5	0	2.0	0	0.5	0	0	0	0	0
10. E.U.	66	M	1.0	0	2.0	0.5	2.0	0.5	2.5	1.5			2.5	0.5	2.0	0	1.0	0
11. J.A.	55	M	0	0	4.0	0.5	5.0	0.5	5.0	1.0			5.0	2.0	4.0	1.0	4.0	1.0
12. D.T.	60	M	0	0.5	1.5	1.0	2.0	1.0					0	0	0	0	0	0
13. V.R.	62	M	1.0	0	1.5	0	2.0	0	2.0	0	2.5	0	1.5	0	1.5	0	1.5	0
14. R.P.	48	M	1.0	0.5	2.0	1.0	2.5	2.0					2.0	1.5	1.0	1.0	0.5	0.5
15. F.Z.	58	F	0	0	1.0	0		0					0	0	0	0	0	0
16. M.L.	45	M																
17. K.Y.S.[a]	56	M	0.5	0	1.0	0	2.5	0		0		0	1.5	0	1.5	0	1.0	0
18. R.C.[a]	35	M	0	0	1.5	0	2.5	0.5		1.0			0.5	0.5	0	0	0	0
19. G.L.[a]	45	F	2.0	1.5	2.0	2.0							1.0	1.5	1.0	1.5	1.0	1.0
20. J.C.	52	M																
21. A.R.	41	M	0	0	0.5	0	1.0	0	1.5	0	1.5		1.5	0	0.5	0	0	0
22. A.R.[a]	43	M	0	0	1.0	0.5	1.5	1.0					1.0	0.5	0	0	0	0
23. C.S.	66	M	1.0	0	2.0	0	3.0	0					2.0	0	1.5	0	1.0	0
24. A.M.S.[b]	41	F	1.5	0	2.0	0	2.5	0	3.0		3.5		2.0	0	1.5	0	1.0	0
$n=$			14	14	14	14	12	13	6	7	4	3	14	14	14	14	14	14
$\underline{Q}=$			0.67	0.42	0.93	0.59	1.11	0.60	1.31	0.64	0.85	0	1.27	0.69	1.11	0.50	1.06	0.37
$\bar{X}=$			0.57	0.17	1.57	0.39	2.25	0.42	2.58	0.5	2.37	0	1.5	0.46	1.03	0.25	0.78	0.17
$p=$			<.05		<.001		<.001		<.05		<.001		<.01		<.05		<.05	

C, Control; N, nifedipine.
[a] Insignificant angiography. [b] Angiography with positive ergonovine test.

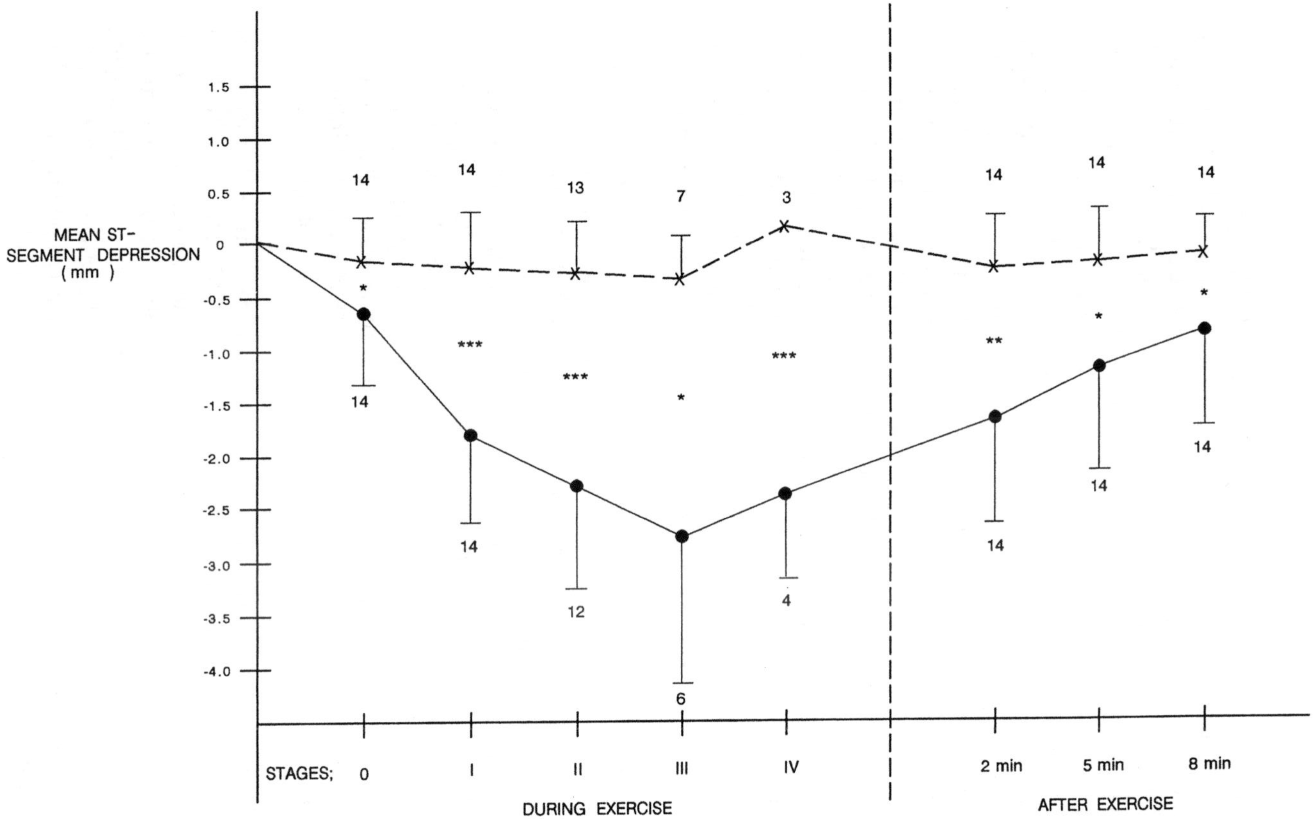

Fig. 1. Mean ST-segment depression changes after nifedipine (X) as compared to control (•). Numbers (above and below the standard-deviation ranges) represent the total number of cases during a particular stage of exercise. *$p<0.05$; **$p<0.01$; ***$p<0.001$

Discussion

Since Feil and Siegel [21] first noted that resting ECG ST-segment depression occurred in patients with angina pectoris, others have observed the similarity of this change in subjects with coronary artery disease during and after exercise [22–24]. Thus, the exercise ECG test became one of the most acceptable noninvasive procedures to confirm coronary insufficiency in anginal cases. Although direct electrode recording of ischemia in the endocardial region produces ST elevation, in the surface ECG the net effect of ST shifting is ST-segment depression. Thus, ST depression may be due to subendocardial ischemia since coronary reserve is exhausted in the subendocardial area ahead of the subepicardial areas and is reflected as ST depression [25–29]. ST depression may also be due to nontransmural ischemia with fixed obstruction pathology with or without vasospasm of epicardial vessels, to subtotal myocardial flow reduction, or to involvement of smaller vessels [30–35]. Animal studies indicate that both epicardial and intramyocardial vessels are responsive to vasoconstrictor stimuli [36]. On exercise an increased rate-pressure product greater than the diastolic pressure time index may result in subendocardial ischemia provided subendocardial coronary reserve is exhausted [37]. As epicardial vessels dilate in response to metabolic demands, coronary pressure distal to a proximal stenosis decrease and may cause hypoperfusion of the subendocardium [38–39].

After myocardial infarction, ST-segment depression detected on exercise testing predicts cardiac deaths within 1 year. Thus, ST depression as a reflection of induceable ischemia warrants cardiac catheterization since these ECG findings help identify high-risk cases or multivessel coronary artery disease [36, 40–47]. Although angina following myocardial infarction with ST depression could also be caused by coronary spasm [48], there is little angiographic evidence that spasm plays a role in postinfarction angina [49–50]. If angiographic findings do not adequately explain patients' symptoms, ergonovine-induced coronary spasm may be seen in postinfarction cases [20]. However, there is reluctance to use ergonovine maleate provocation in postinfarction patients for fear of unresponsiveness of ergonovine-induced spasm to nitroglycerin [51].

T-201 is useful in diagnosing the presence of coronary artery disease but is questionable in distinguishing intramural disease [52–55]. However, thallium defects outside the region of infarct can reliably predict high risk for coronary artery disease [56]. Thallium redistribution scintigraphy also predicts response to coronary bypass surgery of asynergic myocardial segments: T-201 imaging is normal in 90% and abnormal in 76% with reversed and irreversible asynergy, respectively [12]. Reversible ischemia on T-201 scintigraphy can also identify viable myocardium supplied by stenotic coronary arteries [57].

Exercise ECG and nuclear examinations have been considered redundant since the anginal state is the justification for angiographic study [58]. Studies show that with increased workload and rate-pressure product greater perfusion abnormalities exist in patients with coronary artery disease [14]. However, our study in both anginal and post infarction cases after nifedipine showed that rate-pressure product and treadmill duration were significantly higher, while thallium scintigraphy was normal in 70% and improved in 30%, and there were significantly reduced ST-segment changes. These findings indicate that mechanisms other than fixed obstructive lesions are present.

Thus, the immediate need for invasive procedures such as coronary arteriography may be delayed or avoided if after drug intervention ST depression is reduced, and reversible exercise-induced ischemia becomes reperfused on repeat T-201 imaging. In fact, in six anginal patients coronary arteriographic findings were insignificant.

Nifedipine induces lower coronary tone [59, 60], prevents spasm [61], and reduces afterload [62, 63]. In spontaneously hypertensive rats nifedipine prevented progression of left ventricular hypertrophy and the decrease in ventricular compliance [64]. Whatever mechanism is involved, certainly the "improved" exercise test and T-201 reperfusion findings after nifedipine may suggest an insignificant and nonsurgically correctable epicardial coronary disease, intramyocardial flow abnormalities, or exercise-induced vasospastic ST-segment changes. Vasospasm was documented in one case in this study.

Limitation of Study

The relatively small number of subjects and the absence of sufficient coronary arteriographic examinations to establish definitely the presence or absence of obstructed epicardial coronary artery disease may be the basis for potential objection to the results of this study. Angiography demonstrates varying degrees of occlusive disease but does not show intramural changes if subendocardial or nontransmural changes are responsible for the exercise-induced ST-segment changes and T-201 hypoperfusion in our study. Thallium scintigraphy may not reflect significant hypoperfusion indicative of an exercise-induced subendocardial ischemia since coronary flow changes may not be sensitive enough to reflect mild but multiple areas of ischemia, due to overlapping of structures, limited resolution of gamma camera, some uncertainties in the timing of isotope injection, and the subsequent dynamic state of the myocardial isotope washin and washout [65]. Flow reduction of 40%–60% are inconsistently detected by qualitative or visual image analysis [66]. Thus, direct vasospasm of intramyocardial vessels cannot be demonstrated by current clinical methods either at rest or at effort. There may be spontaneous changes in myocardial perfusion imaging because of progressive development of collateral circulation, which could occur within 3 months after myocardial infarction [67, 68]. Our postinfarction cases were studied more than 3 months after the acute episode.

Vasoactive component cannot be ruled out and is difficult to prove in the anginal syndrome with ST-segment depression at rest or on exercise testing despite demonstration on coronary arteriography of significant occlusive disease [69]. This is particularly so in patients who on mild effort or emotional upsets develop angina plus the demonstration of incurred epicardial coronary vasomotor tone in association with existing atherosclerotic luminal narrowing which may diminish vasodilatory reserve [70].

The assumption is that a normal T-201 scintigraphy negates significant coronary flow reduction. After drug intervention, nifedipine may have counteracted the vasospastic mechanisms in both epicardial (as demonstrated in patient 24) and intramyocardial vessels. With afterload reduction, wall stress is reduced, and endocardial coronary flow may increase. Despite a possible demonstration of epicardial occlusive disease intramural flow improvement cannot be excluded. Thus, in six of these cases coronary arteriography showed insignificant epicardial fixed obstructive disease.

A prospective study with more cases is desirable. Any angina or postinfarction case with "ischemic ST segment" and reversible T-201 hypoperfused area may require a calcium antagonist such as nifedipine to determine the dynamic or fixed status of the exercise-induced ischemia. The need for, and risk with, coronary arteriography may be avoided if after calcium blockers exercise-induced ischemic areas become reperfused.

Acknowledgements: Thallium imaging was done at the Philippine Heart Center for Asia. Thallium imaging interpretations were given independently by Drs. Eduardo Villacorta and Emiliano Ramos.

References

1. Cannon PJ, Schmidt DH, Weiss MB et al. (1975) The relationship between regional myocardial perfusion at rest and arteriographic lesions in patients with coronary arteriosclerosis. J Clin Invest 56:1442
2. Klocke FJ, Bunnel IL, Greene DG, Wittenberg SM, Visco JP (1974) Average coronary blood flow per unit weight of left ventricle in patients with and without coronary artery disease. Circulation 50:547
3. Gould KL, Lipscomb K, Hamilton GW (1974) Physiologic basis for assessing critical coronary stenosis. Instantaneous flow response and regional distribution during coronary hyperemia as measures of coronary flow reserve. Am J Cardiol 33:87
4. Gould KL, Lipscomb K (1974) Effects of coronary stenosis on coronary flow reserve and resistance. Am J Cardiol 34:48
5. Brandi G, McGregor M (1969) Intramural pressure in the left ventricle of the dog. Cardiovasc Res 3:472
6. Baird R, Mantelow R, Shah P, Amili FM (1970) Intramyocardial pressure - study of regional variations and its relationship to intraventricular pressure. J Thorac Cardiovasc Surg 5:810
7. Levin DC (1974) Pathways and functional significance of the coronary collateral circulation. Circulation 50:831
8. Hamby RI, Aintablian A, Schwartz A (1976) Reappraisal of the functional significance of the coronary collateral circulation. Am J Cardiol 38:305
9. Baroldi G (1973) Coronary heart disease significance of the morphologic lesions. Am Heart J 85:1
10. Hammermeister KE, Kennedy JW, Hamilton GW et al. (1974) Aortocoronary saphenous vein bypass; failure of successful grafting to improve resting left ventricular function in chronic angina. N Engl J Med 290:186

11. Mintz LJ, Ingels NB, Daughters GT II, Stinson EB, Alderman EL (1980) Sequential studies of left ventricular function and wall motion after coronary arterial bypass surgery. Am J Cardiol 45:210
12. Rozanski A, Berman DS, Gray R et al. (1981) Use of thallium 201 redistribution scintigraphy in the preoperative differentiation of reversible and non-reversible myocardial asynergy. Circulation 64:936
13. Mock MB, Ringquist I, Fisher LD, Davis KB et al. (1982) Survival of medically treated patients in the coronary artery surgery study (CASS) registry. Circulation 66:562
14. McLaughlin PR, Martin RP, Doherty P et al. (1977) Reproducibility of thallium 201 myocardial imaging. Circulation 55:497
15. Sanmarco ME, Pontius S, Selvester RH (1980) Abnormal blood pressure response and marked ischemic ST-segment depression as predictors of severe coronary artery disease. Circulation 61:572
16. Bartel AG, Behar VS, Peter RH, Orgain ES, Kong Y (1974) Graded exercise stress tests in angiographically documented coronary artery disease. Circulation 49:348
17. Cheitlin MD, David JE, Castro CM, Barrow EA, Anderson WT (1975) Correlations of "critical" left coronary artery lesions with positive submaximal exercise tests in patients with chest pain. Am Heart J 89:305
18. Kramer N, Susmand A, Shekelle RB (1978) The false negative treadmill exercise test and left ventricular dysfunction. Circulation 57:763
19. Goldman S, Tselos S, Cohn K (1976) Marked depth of ST-segment depression during treadmill exercise testing. Chest 69:729
20. Moran TJ, French WJ, Abrams HF, Criley JM (1982) Postmyocardial infarction angina and coronary spasm. Am J Cardiol 50:197
21. Feil H, Siegel MI (1928) Electrocardiographic changes during attacks of angina pectoris. Am J Med Sci 175:255
22. Wood FN, Wolferth CC (1931) Angina pectoris. The clinical and electrocardiographic phenomena of the attack and their comparison with the effects of experimental temporary coronary occlusion. Arch Intern Med 47:339
23. Wilson FN, Johnston FD (1941) The occurrence in angina pectoris of electrocardiographic changes similar in magnitude and kind to those produced by myocardial infarction. Am Heart J 22:64
24. Abarquez RF jr, Freiman AH, Reichel F, LaDue JS (1960) The precordial electrocardiogram during exercise. Circulation 22:1060
25. Moran LG, Flowers NC (1980) Electrocardiography and vectocardiography. In: Braunwald E (ed) Heart disease. W. B. Saunders, Philadelphia, p 231
26. Guyton RA, McClenathan JH, Newman GE, Michaels LL (1977) Significance of subendocardial ST-segment elevation caused by coronary stenosis in the dog. Am J Cardiol 40:373
27. Weintraub WS, Hattori S, Agarwal JB, Bodenheimer MM, Banka VS, Helfant RH (1981) The relationship between myocardial blood flow and contraction by myocardial layer in the canine left ventricle during ischemia. Circ Res 48:430
28. Weintraub WS, Hattori S, Agarwal J, Bodenheimer MM, Banka VS, Helfant RH (1981) Variable effect of nifedipine on myocardial blood flow at three grades of coronary occlusion in the dog. Circ Res 48:937
29. Rouleau J, Boerboom LE, Surjadhana A, Hoffman JIE (1979) The role of autoregulation and tissue diastolic pressures in the transmural distribution of left ventricular blood flow in anesthetized dogs. Circ Res 45:804
30. Weiner L, Kasparian H, Duca PR et al. (1976) Spectrum of coronary arterial spasm. Clinical angiographic and myocardial metabolic experience in 29 cases. Am J Cardiol 38:945
31. Helfant RH (1979) Coronary spasm. Am J Cardiol 44:839
32. Tri TB, Price HL, Sobol SM (1982) Nifedipine therapy for small vessel disease of the heart. Am J Cardiol 50:211
33. Pepine CJ, Feldmars RL, Conti CR (1980) Observations on the role of coronary artery spasm in stress induced angina. Circulation 62 [Suppl III]:312

34. Waters DD, Szlachcic J, Theroux P, Dauwe F, Mizgala HF (1981) Ergonovine testing to detect spontaneous remissions of angina during long term treatment with calcium antagonist drugs. Am J Cardiol 47:179
35. Hempler FA jr, Proudfit WL, Razadi M, Shirly EK, Greenstreet R, Sheldon WC (1978) Ergonovine maleate provocative test for coronary arterial spasm. Am J Cardiol 41:631
36. Epstein SF, Palmeri ST, Patterson RE (1982) Evaluation of patients after acute myocardial infarction. Indications for cardiac catheterization and surgical intervention. N Engl J Med 307:1487
37. Frazier J, Cooper N, Buckberg G (1974) The adequacy of subendocardial oxygen delivery; the interaction of determinants of low arterial oxygen content and myocardial oxygen need. Circulation 49:968
38. Mair TW (1972) Subendocardial distribution of coronary blood flow and the effect of antianginal drugs. Circ Res 30:621
39. Lipscomb K, Gould KL (1975) Mechanism of the effect of coronary artery stenosis on coronary flow in the dog. Am Heart J 89:60
40. Kavanagh T, Shepard RJ, Chisholn AW, Quereshi S, Kennedy J (1979) Prognostic indexes for patients with ischemic heart disease enrolled in an exercise-centered rehabilitation program. Am J Cardiol 44:1225
41. Sami H, Kraemer H, Debusk RF (1979) The prognostic significance of serial exercise testing after myocardial infarction. Circulation 60:1238
42. Theroux P, Waters DD, Halyhen C, Debalsieux JS, Mizgala HR (1979) Prognostic value of exercise testing soon after myocardial infarction. N Engl J Med 301:341
43. Weiner DA, McCabe C, Lein MD, Ryan TJ (1978) ST-segment change post infarction: predictive value for multivessel coronary disease and left ventricular aneurysm. Circulation 58:887
44. Castellanet MJ, Greenberg PS, Ellestad MH (1978) Comparison of ST-segment changes on exercise testing with angiographic findings in patients with prior myocardial infarction. Am J Cardiol 42:29
45. Chaitman BR, Waters DD, Corgara F, Bourassa MG (1978) Prediction of multivessel disease after inferior myocardial infarction. Circulation 57:1085
46. Morris SN, McHenry RL (1978) Role of exercise stress testing in healthy subjects in patients with coronary artery disease. Controversies in cardiology. Am J Cardiol 42:659
47. Cohn K, Kamm B, Fetcih N, Brand R, Goldschlager N (1979) Use of treadmill score to quantify response and predict extent of coronary disease. Circulation 59:286
48. Koiwaya Y, Torri S, Takeshita A, Nakagaki O, Nakamura M (1982) Post-infarction angina caused by coronary arterial spasm. Circulation 65:275
49. Johnson AD, Deteviler JH (1979) Coronary spasm, variant angina and recurrent myocardial infarction. Circulation 59:297
50. King SB, Mansour KA, Hatcher CR, Silverman ME, Hart NC (1973) Coronary spasm producing Prinzmetal's angina and myocardial infarction in the absence of coronary atherosclerosis. Am Thorac Surg 16:337
51. Madias JE (1979) The syndrome of variant angina culminating in acute myocardial infarction. Circulation 59:297
52. Ritchie J, Trobaugh G, Hamilton G et al. (1977) Myocardial imaging with thallium 201 at rest and during exercise: comparison with coronary arteriography and resting exercise ECG. Circulation 56:66
53. Zaret BL (1977) Myocardial imaging with radioactive potassium and its analogs. Prog Cardiovasc Dis 20:81
54. Dash H, Massie BM, Bolvinick EH, Brundage BH (1979) The non-invasive identification of left main and three-vessel coronary artery disease by myocardial stress perfusion, scintigraphy and treadmill exercise electrocardiography. Circulation 60:276
55. Massie BM, Bolvinick EH, Brundage BH (1979) Correlation of thallium 201 scintigrams with coronary anatomy; factors affecting region sensitivity. Am J Cardiol 44:616

56. Patterson RE, Horowitz SF, Eng C et al. (1983) Can non-invasive exercise test criteria identify patients with left main or three-vessel coronary disease after a first myocardial infarction? Am J Cardiol 51:361
57. Turner JD, Schwartz KW, Logic JR et al. (1980) Detection of residual jeopardized myocardium 3 weeks after myocardial infarction by exercise testing with thallium 201 myocardial scintigraphy. Circulation 61:729
58. Freisinger GC (1982) The reasonable workup before recommending medical or surgical therapy: an overall strategy. Circulation 65 (II):21
59. Gunther S, Green L, Muller JE, Mudge GH jr, Grossman W (1979) Inappropriate coronary vasoconstriction in patients with coronary artery disease: a role for nifedipine. Am J Cardiol 44:793
60. De Servi S, Mussini A, Specchia G et al. (1980) Effects of nifedipine on coronary blood flow, coronary resistance during cold pressor test and isometric exercise in patients with coronary artery disease. Am Heart J 1 [Suppl D]:43
61. Freedman B, Dunn RF, Richmond DR, Kelly DT (1981) Coronary artery spasm during exercise; treatment with verapamil. Circulation 64:68
62. Moskowitz RM, Piccini TA, Nacarelli GV, Zellis R (1979) Nifedipine therapy for stable angina pectoris: preliminary results of effects on angina frequency and treadmill exercise response. Am J Cardiol 44:811
63. Kallenback M, Schultz W, Kober G (1979) Effects of nifedipine after intravenous and intra-coronary administration. Am J Cardiol 44:832
64. Motz W, Strauer BE (1983) The influence of nifedipine on LV compliance and myocardial stiffness. J Am Coll Cardiol 1(2):1641
65. Ritchie JL (1982) Myocardial perfusion imaging. Am J Cardiol 49:1341
66. Mueller TM, Marcus ML, Ehrhardt JC, Chaudhurt T, Abboud FM (1976) Limitations of thallium 201 myocardial perfusion scintigrams. Circulation 54:640
67. Dorer JS, Rosing DR, Miller RM et al. (1980) Natural history of left ventricular function during one year after acute myocardial infarction: comparison with clinical electrocardiographic and biochemical determinations. Am J Cardiol 46:1
68. Buda AJ, Dubbin JD, MacDonald IL, Straus HD, Orr SA, Meindok H (1982) Spontaneous changes in thallium 201 myocardial perfusion imaging after myocardial infarction. Am J Cardiol 50:1272
69. Brown G (1981) Coronary spasm observations linking the clinical spectrum of ischemic heart disease to the dynamic pathology of coronary atherosclerosis. Arch Intern Med 141:716
70. Maseri A, Pesola A, Marzilli M et al. (1977) Coronary vasospasm in angina pectoris. Lancet i:713

Newest Information on Unstable Angina Pectoris

P. G. Hugenholtz[1]

Introduction

The clinical syndrome of unstable angina continues to excite and confuse the clinician. This is largely because of the difficulties in marking the exact "watershed" between angina (a potentially reversible form of ischemia) and myocardial infarction (after 30 min an irreversible process; Table 1). Deciding in which state of ischemia a patient finds himself belongs to the most difficult decisions to be made in clinical medicine.

While it is true that not every case of unstable angina leads to myocardial infarction or sudden death, it is also evident that in most individuals some symptoms or signs of the unstable angina sydrome have actually preceded the irreversible event. The difficulty lies in the accurate recognition of the watershed. Despite intense efforts over the past two decades to elucidate the exact pathophysiology, an accurate understanding of the natural history in a given patient, whether in or outside of hospital, remains extremely difficult. It is this uncertainty of outcome in a given patient which obliges the physician to attack several factors in the perceived causation of the syndrome at the same time without clear knowledge as to which is the dominant one. As Balakumaran et al. [1] have succinctly put it:

> Unstable angina is doubly distressing. On the one hand the patient is confronted with the disturbing new symptomatology, namely unfamiliar pain (crescendo angina), unprovoked pain (angina at rest) or pain returning on the heels on the major blow of myocardial infarction (early postinfarct angina), on the other hand the physician knows that something potentially dangerous is afoot.

Recently two further findings have helped to fill in the puzzle. One is a paper from the Netherlands reporting on a medium-sized multicenter randomized trial evaluating the usefulness of a calcium antagonist (nifedipine), a β-blocker (metoprolol), and their combined use versus placebo. The other paper, one from California by Sherman et al. [2], presents a marvel of diagnostic information since by means of a miniature intra-arterial fiber optic technique

---

[1] Thoraxcenter, Department of Cardiology, University Hospital, Erasmus University Rotterdam, The Netherlands

the actual lesion causing the unstable angina syndrome is literally brought into cardiovascular focus. This information, coupled with that presented earlier by Falk et al. [3] and Davies and Thomas [4], has drastically altered our concept of the pathophysiology underlying the unstable angina syndrome. While a decade ago spasm was considered a leading contender as the cause of the unstable state, current evidence points toward the ruptured plaque with superimposed thrombus, also an intermittent phenomenon, as the most likely explanation. A third piece of the puzzle was provided by the paper of De Feyter et al. [5], also from the Netherlands, which in therapeutic terms confirms the concept that non-spasm-induced obstruction of the coronary blood supply is most often at the root of the problem and must be solved by mechanical means at an early stage when drugs prove no early relief.

Pathophysiology

Patients with unstable angina, in contrast to those with stable angina, are a widely heterogeneous group of patients with varying degrees of coronary atherosclerosis, varying chances of sudden plaque rupture, and the presence of (in)complete degrees of (intermittent) thrombosis (Fig. 1). In addition, there is to varying degrees the associated impairment of left ventricular function, which makes the interpretation of clinical symptoms even more complex. Many authors, such as Maseri and Foale [6], Conti [7], Julian [8], and Hugenholtz et al. [9] have detailed the changing concepts over the past decades.

The pathophysiologic confusion alluded to above begins with the definition. Some clinicians accept the definition proposed more than 10 years ago by Conti [7] that reserves the term unstable angina for patients who are observed to have an anginal attack, with coincident electrocardiographic changes such as T-wave inversion and ST-segment elevation, but without at-

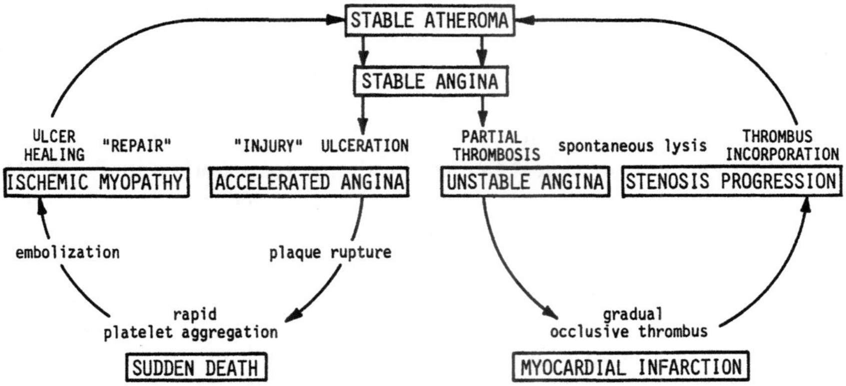

Fig. 1. The ulceration-thrombosis cycle of coronary disease. (From [3, 4])

tendant enzyme release. Such pain attacks must last at least 15 min and should be associated with the usual signs of ischemia of the myocardium with attendant instability of the cardiovascular state (e.g., tachycardia, blood pressure decline). Others, such as those designing the HINT trial [10] felt that the diagnosis should be widened to include patients who had had one or more attacks of unstable angina in the 12 h preceding admission. It is generally known, however, that such historical evidence may be misleading and, as is evident from the HINT trial [10], may actually reflect an (incompletely remembered) attack of pain reflecting myocardial infarction. These attacks do not constitute actual unstable angina, for the essence of the latter diagnosis is that there is still viable tissue "to go after."

The significant and essential requirement, therfore, to identify "real" unstable angina is that the pain is present, continuing, or even progressive in severity and intensity despite bedrest. If, as has recently become evident from various arteriographic studies [11-13], such "invasive" observations are made immediately after, or even during, the attack of unstable angina, quite a different anatomic picture emerges. Rather then spasm, thrombus is visualized on top of the fractured atherosclerotic lesion. The paper by Sherman et al. [2] alluded to above confirms this by direct visual inspection. From the above data it becomes clear that "real" unstable angina, as defined by the Conti criteria [9], more often than not requires a nonpharmacological approach which should be aimed at opening up the vessel by mechanical means such as a percutaneously introduced balloon catheter, by cardiovascular surgery, or by a thrombolytic approach with an effective agent in combination with the first. Clearly, such patients were not included in the HINT study [10] which, as the authors point out in their paper, consisted only of patients who had had a history of an attack of angina pectoris within the 12 h preceding admission, or who were observed to have such an attack while in the hospital but which was seen to respond to nitroglycerin or other efforts at pain relief. Those with persistent pain despite these efforts were excluded, in fact eliminating the majority of patients with "real" unstable angina from the study.

The stated aim of that study was to determine whether in the remaining group of patients the pharmacological approach could avoid the subsequent occurrence of ischemia or myocardial infarction. It is therefore clear that this form of unstable angina is a much milder one than the high-risk group seen by De Feyter et al. [5] and visualized in the studies by Sherman et al. [2]. It therefore also becomes clear that the kind of patient studied in the HINT trial [10] corresponds much more to that recently reported upon by Mulcahy et al. [14], who found in 1 year a 14% myocardial infarction rate and a 1-year mortality rate of 8%. Unfortunately, the HINT trial [10] provides no long-term mortality or morbidity data. Even so, the 48-h morbidity data in the placebo group consisting of 84 patients, most of whom were classified retrospectively as belonging to the low- or medium-risk group, showed myocardial infarction within 48 h in 13 (15%) and a definite myocardial infarction with onset of Q-waves within 48 h of 11%. Thus, this kind of patient fits the Mulcahy et al.

[14] type of observation. Also in the Mulcahy et al. observation the patients were not included until a 24-h observation period had elapsed, during which presumably the more severe patients were sent on for more definitive therapy.

It is of interest to note while the HINT trial [10] in the Netherlands was proceeding between 1981 and 1984, the paper by De Feyter et al. [5] appeared covering experiences in one of the participating hospitals for the more severe type of unstable angina, the one corresponding to the definition by Conti [7]. These patients, none of whom had responded to triple pharmacological therapy observed for at least 24 h, usually arrived in the cardiac catheterization laboratory with pain, and most underwent percutaneous TCA as an emergency procedure. It is striking to note that despite the severe form of obstruction and attendant ischemia, excellent results were obtained as soon as the vessel was deobstructed with no procedure-related mortality, one delayed sudden death (at 6 months), and a 1-year myocardial infarction rate either from the procedure or subsequent to the procedure of only 6%.

It now becomes clear that the real issue in the management of patients with varying forms of unstable angina does not lie in the availability of appropriate treatment but in the nonavailability of adequate diagnostic procedures. As the authors of the HINT trial [10] observe, "These results show that it is impossible to delineate reversible ischemia (i.e. unstable angina) reliably from irreversible ischemia (i.e. myocardial infarction) early on clinical grounds". In fact, the myocardial infarction rate for the placebo group study was at best 15%, and if Q-waves are not required, 11%. It is appropriate therefore once more to review the time sequence of events that may occur immediately after the onset of angina pectoris.

Timing of Intervention

Recent studies from our laboratory [15] have demonstrated that during balloon dilatation of a human coronary artery, complete occlusion of up to 5 min can be tolerated without permanent metabolic defect or severe angina, although already within 10–20 s potassium and lactate levels in the coronary sinus efflux increase dramatically, indicating altered O_2-dependent metabolism. Shortly thereafter breakdown products of the high-energy phosphate metabolism such as inosine and hypoxanthine appear in the efflux of the coronary circulation. Such biochemical markers of ischemia denote initially a temporary metabolic disruption but presage the onset of ECG changes and of cellular destruction which begins in the 15th min [16]. These metabolic and electric abnormalities precede other signs of ischemia such as changed mechanical performance of the heart, e.g., loss of diastolic tone and impaired relaxation, as well as enzyme release, arrhythmias, and eventually anginal pain (Table 1).

Table 1. Time scale of events in myocardial ischemia

Metabolic activity (release of H^+, K^+, etc.)	0–10 s
Left ventricular dysfunction/E-C coupling	20 s
Fall in creatine phosphate	20 s
ECG changes, T-wave, ST-segment	30 s
Chest pain (cave "silent" episodes)	60 s
Release of vasoactive substances	60 s
Increased sympathetic activity	0–60 s
Fall in ATP levels	2 min
Irreversible damage in core	15 min
Ultrastructural changes	20 min
Malfunction of mitochondria	40 min
Malfunction of sarcoplasmic reticulum (Ca^{2+} transport)	40 min

Other clinical observations from our laboratory [17] have shown that even when successful thrombolysis is achieved within 30 min after the onset of symptoms, some degree of irreversible myocardial damage has already occurred in the core of the ischemic area. Thus, in the setting of the syndrome of unstable angina time intervals gain major importance. In this regard, the concept of a significant borderzone, marginally perfused but susceptible to manipulation by interventions, must be discussed. Hearse and associates [16] have indicated that three distinct states of reduced flow and ischemic injury may coexist, and that they determine the practicability of tissue salvage. These researchers distinguish among "tolerable," "critical," and "lethal" ischemia.

In "tolerable" ischemia flow reduction of up to 50% may exist, and tissue energy stores are hardly depleted. It appears that many of the patients in the HINT study [10] were in fact in this category. Here the vasodilator characteristic of calcium antagonist therapy and the blockade of excessive adrenergic substances by β-blockers appears the best therapy, preferably in combination.

In "critical" ischemia flow is reduced by as much as 80%, intracellular energy levels become rapidly reduced, and tissue is jeopardized within minutes. Only timely (30 min to 4 h) reperfusion efforts may lead to salvage of the tissue. This seems to be the kind of patient described by De Feyter et al. [5] and visualized by Sherman et al. [2]. In this category ultimately a combination of thrombolytic therapy with percutaneous TCA and/or bypass grafting seems mandatory, with pharmacological therapy being relegated to secondary place.

In "lethal" ischemia, in which flow reduction exceeds 80%, and tissue energy stores are very rapidly depleted, tissue is certain to die even earlier. Such patients have a severe plaque rupture, rapidly expanding in volume and occluding the vessel within a matter of minutes rather than hours with or without superimposed thrombus. From the recently published Netherlands Interuniversity Cardiology Trial on Streptokinase [18], in which 533 patients with acute myocardial infarction were randomized either to conventional therapy in the coronary care unit or to early thrombolytic therapy with streptokinase, the results in the subset treated with intravenous streptokinase within 90 min of onset of symptoms and followed by deobstruction by means of intracoronary streptokinase and/or percutaneous TCA, substantiated the possibility that complete reperfusion provides major benefit. A 1-year mortality of only 2% was seen in this subset versus one of 16% in the randomized controls. Furthermore, it was shown that in the larger group of patients who received lytic therapy within 2 h of the onset of symptoms, infarct size was limited by up to 40%, and ventricular function preserved (average ejection fraction, 53%). Furthermore, in this group a 50% reduction of mortality relative to the conventionally treated patients was obtained [18].

This type of division into tolerable, critical, and lethal forms of ischemia, although difficult to detect clinically with the present methodology, is mandatory for proper interpretation of the results reported in the HINT trial [10]. Thus, it is not surprising that in the group of patients who entered the trial without prior β-blockade after exclusion of those with persistent severe symptoms, no difference was found between placebo, metoprolol, and the combination of metoprolol and nifedipine. All had such mild forms of the disease (only 87 of 333 were in the high-risk group) that spontaneous improvement of the "tolerable" ischemia could occur. It is not clear why in this same group of patients not pretreated with a β-blocker, nifedipine monotherapy increased the risk of progression to myocardial infarction. Apart from its being a chance finding, the most likely explanation appears to be uncertainty as to when the onset of myocardial infarction took place. Furthermore, the increased number of high-risk patients (46 in the nifedipine group versus 7 with metoprolol and 14 with placebo) seems to be "loading" the nifedipine group disproportionally. Also, the wide time intervals in enzyme assessment and the known unreliability of enzyme release in accurately assessing the onset of myocardial infarction with the infrequent sampling rate suggest that there was a disproportional number of patients who either sustained their infarct immediately preceding (or at the time of) inclusion into the trial. If so, these findings confirm reports from other trials with nifedipine in myocardial infarction which have shown that neither this [19, 20] nor any other calcium antagonist [21] can alter the events once necrosis has taken place. In fact, these drugs are markedly ineffective under such circumstances, while they are quite effective in early unstable angine (Table 2) [22–24]. On the other hand, in the group of 177 patients out of the 527 who did receive β-blocker therapy prior to admission, the addition of nifedipine was not detrimental. It actually showed a reduction in complications as high as that shown by the combination of metoprolol with nifedipine in the 1982 trial by Gerstenblith et al. [25].

In summary, the appropriate therapies for unstable angina (Fig. 2) depend primarily on the adequate assessment of the state of cardiac derangement. Early ischemia with vasoconstriction without significant obstruction reacts to double or triple pharmacotherapy; protracted ischemia and nearly complete obstruction of a major nutrient vessel requires prompt revascularization. It remains the difficult task of the specialist to choose the correct approach.

Table 2. Potential indications for use of Ca^{2+} antagonists as "cardioprotective" in pre- or re-ischemic states on clinical and experimental grounds

1) Unstable angina with signs of "tolerable" ischemia (by ECG, echo, thallium, or biochemical markers)
2) Within 0–3 h after onset of symptoms and signs of myocardial ischemia
3) During post-infarction recurent ischemia
4) When "stunned" myocardium is suspected (repeated brief ischemic attacks, "crescendo angina")
5) Prophylactically after sustained infarction when residual stenoses are suspected
6) During intentional disturbance of coronary perfusion CA, aorta cross-clamping during coronary surgery)
7) During thrombolytic therapy of coronary obstruction, provided the latter is carried out within 0–4 h after onset of symptoms
8) When rapid afterload reduction seems advisable with a β-blocker to avoid reflex tachycardia
9) Prophylactically when recurrent spasm as a cause of ischemia is anticipated in Prinzmetal's variant angina, intracoronary manipulation such as PTCA, etc.

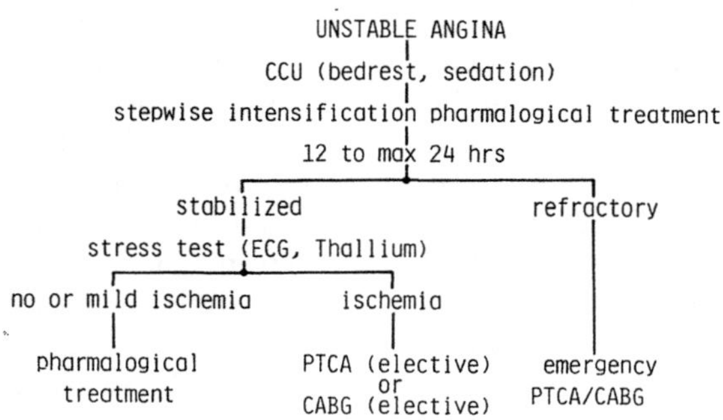

Fig. 2. Proposed management of patients with unstable angina: persistent chest pain at rest associated with electrocardiographic changes

References

1. Balakumaran K, Fioretti P, Brower RW et al. (1985) Unstable angina und myocardial revascularisation. In: Hugenholtz PG, Goldman BS (eds) Unstable angina, current concepts and management. Schattauer, Stuttgart, pp 309–317
2. Sherman CT, Litvack F, Grundvert W (1986) Coronary angioscopy in patients with unstable angina pectoris. N Engl M 315:913–919
3. Falk E (1985) Unstable angina with fetal outcome: dynamic coronary thrombosis leading to infarction and/or sudden death. Circulation 71:699–708
4. Davies MJ, Thomas A (1984) Thrombosis and acute coronary artery lesions in sudden cardiac ischemic death. N Engl J Med 310:1137–1140
5. de Feyter PJ, Serruys PW, van den Brand M et al. (1985) Emergency coronary angioplasty in refractory unstable angina. N Engl J Med 313:342–346
6. Maseri A, Foale R (1985) A pathophysiological classification of unstable angina. In: Hugenholtz PG, Goldman BS (eds) Unstable angina, current concepts and management. Schattauer, Stuttgart, pp 71–78
7. Conti CR (1985) Unstable angina: thoughts on pathogenesis. In: Hugenholtz PG, Goldman BS (eds) Unstable angina, current concepts and management. Stuttgart, pp 55–64

8. Julian DG (1985) The natural history of unstable angina. In: Hugenholtz PG, Goldman BS (eds) Unstable angina, current concepts and management. Schattauer, Stuttgart, pp 65–70
9. Hugenholtz PG, Goldman BS (eds) (1985) Unstable angina, current concepts and management. Schattauer, Stuttgart, pp 1–10
10. Lubsen J, Thijssen JGP, Kerkkamp HJJ et al. (1986) Report of the Holland Interuniversity nifedipine-metoprolol Trial (HINT research group). Early treatment of unstable angina at the coronary care unit: a randomized, double blind, placebo controlled comparison of recurrent ischaemia in patients with nifedipine and/or metoprolol. Br Heart J 56:400–413
11. Cowley MJ, Disciascio G, Vetrovec GW (1985) Coronary thrombus in unstable angina: angiographic observation and clinical relevance. In: Hugenholtz PG, Goldman BS (eds) Unstable angina, current concepts and management. Schattauer, Stuttgart, 95–102
12. Bresnahan DR, Davis JL, Homes DR jr et al. (1985) Angiographic occurrence and clinical correlates of intraluminal coronary artery thrombus: role of unstable angina. J Am Coll Cardiol 6:285–289
13. Zack PM, Ischinger T, Aker UT et al. (1984) The occurrence of angiograhically detected intracoronary thrombus in patients with unstable angina pectoris. Am Heart J 108:1408–1411
14. Mulcahy R, Al Awadhi AH, de Buitleon M (1985) Natural history and prognosis of unstable angina. Am Heart J 109:753–758
15. Serruys PW, Wijns W, van den Brand M et al. (1984) Left ventricular performance, regional blood flow, wall motion and lactate metabolism during transluminal angioplasty. Circulation 70:25–36
16. Verdouw PD, Hartog JM, Saxena PR, Hugenholtz PG (1986) Systematic and regional hemodynamic, antiarrhythmic and antiischemic effects of berantolol in anesthesized pigs. Am J Cardiol 58:8E–16E
17. Serruys PW, Simoons ML, Suryapranata H et al. (1986) Preservation of global and regional left ventricular function after early thrombolysis in acute myocardial infarction. J Am Coll Cardiol 7:729–742
18. Simoons MS, Serruys PW, van den Brand M et al. (1985) Improved survival after early thrombolysis in acute myocardial infarction. A randomized trial conducted by the Interuniversity Cardiology Institute in the Netherlands. Lancet ii 578–582
19. Hugenholtz PG, Serruys PW, Fleckenstein A et al. (1986) Why Ca^{2+} antagonists will be most useful before or during early myocardial ischemia and not after infarction has been established. Eur Heart J 7:270–278
20. Sirnes PA, Overskeid K, Pedersen TR, Bathen J, Drivenes A, Frøland Gs, Kjekshus JK, Landmark K, Rokseth R, Sirnes KE, Sundøy A, Torjussen BR, Westlund KM, Wik BA (1984) The Norwegian Nifedipine Multicenter Trial. Circulation 70:638–644
21. Hansen JF, Sigurd B, Mellemgard K, Lyngbye J (1980) Verapamil in acute myocardial infarction. Clin Invest Med 3:159–163
22. Muller JE, Turi ZG, Pearle DL, Schneider JF, Serfas DH, Morrison J, Stone PH, Rude RE, Rosner B, Sobel BE, Tate C, Schneider E, Roberts R, Hennekens CH, Braunwald E (1984) Nifedipine and conventional therapy for unstable angina pectoris: a randomized double-blind comparison. Circulation 69:728–739
23. Nayler WG, Ferrari R, Williams A (1980) Protective effect of pretreatment with verapamil, nifedipine and propranolol on mitochondrial function in the ischemic and reperfused myocardium. Am J Cardiol 46:242–248
24. Verdouw PD, Essed CE, Hugenholtz PG, Lamers JMJ (1985) On the role of Ca^{2+} slow channel blockers in the treatment of myocardial ischemia. In: Hugenholtz PG, Goldman BS (eds) Unstable angina, current concepts and management. Schattauer, Stuttgart, pp 177–186
25. Gerstenblith G, Ouyang P, Achuff SC, Bulkley BH, Becker LC, Mellits ED, Baughman KL, Weiss JL, Flaherty JT, Kolman CH, Llewellyn M, Weisfeld ML (1982) Nifedipine in unstable angina: a double blind randomized trial. N Engl J Med 306:885–894

Effect of Nifedipine on Relaxation and Early Left Ventricular Filling During Postpacing Ischemic Period

Y. Nakamura[1], S. Sasayama[2], H. Nonogi[1], S. Miyazaki[1], Y. Kihara[1], T. Konishi[1], and C. Kawai[1]

Introduction

Nifedipine has been shown to improve left ventricular performance during ischemia (Emanuelsson and Holmberg 1983; Lorell et al. 1981; Nelson et al. 1984; Tiefenbrunn et al. 1983). Although it has been reported that nifedipine can improve diastolic properties of hypertrophic cardiomyopathy (Lorell et al. 1982), whether it can modify relaxation and ventricular filling abnormalities during ischemia is not yet know. Since left ventricular relaxation and filling are important functions for ventricular ejection, which comes next in the cardiac cycle, we studied the effects of nifedipine on relaxation and early ventricular filling in patients with coronary artery disease during postpacing ischemic periods.

Methods

Study Patients

Our six patients (five women and one man) were aged 44–71 years and had effort-induced angina pectoris. None had had a prior myocardial infarction, and patients with unstable angina or acute myocardial infarction were excluded. All patients were in sinus rhythm. Informed consent was obtained.

Catheterization and Cineangiography

Premedication consisted of 5 mg diazepam orally 1 h before cardiac catheterization. All medications were withheld for at least 12 h before the procedure. Catheterization was performed via the brachial approach. After routine right heart catheterization with a Swan-Ganz catheter and left heart catheterization with a Sones catheter, coronary arteriography was performed by the Sones

[1] Third Dept. of Internal Medicine, Faculty of Medicine, Kyoto University, Kyoto, Japan
[2] Second Dept. of Medicine, Toyama Medical and Pharmaceutical University, Faculty of Medicine, Toyama, Japan

technique. A pacing catheter was then positioned in the right atrium and a high fidelity micromanometer-tipped angiocatheter (Mikro-tip, model PC-481, Millar Instruments) was introduced into the left ventricle. Baseline drift was checked by comparison with a Statham P23Db transducer connected to the catheter's fluid-filled lumen for angiography. The zero level of the fluid system was set at the midchest position. When it was confirmed that ventricular pressure had returned to baseline after coronary arteriography, left ventricular cineangiography was performed in the 30° right anterior oblique projection with a Phillips 9-in. image intensification system. Left ventricular opacification was achieved by injecting 25–35 ml radiopaque contrast medium (80% Angiografin) through the catheter at a rate of 12 ml/s. Films were exposed at a rate of 60 frames/s with an Ari 35-mm cine camera. High-fidelity left ventricular pressure, electrocardiogram, cineangiographic frame markers, and an injection marker were simultaneously recorded at a paper speed of 100 mm/s with a multichannel optical recording system (VR-12 Simultrace Recorder, Electronics for Medicine). Two lead markers were placed on the image itensifier as fixed external references for superimposition of the images.

Pacing Protocol

Atrial pacing was initiated at a rate of 90 beats/min and was increased in increments of 30 beats/min every 2 min. In patients in whom atrioventricular block developed during atrial pacing, right ventricular pacing was substituted. Pacing was stopped with the occurrence of chest pain. If well tolerated, pacing was continued at a rate of 150 beats/min for 6 min. Therefore, the maximum total duration of pacing was 10 min (i.e., 90 beats/min for 2 min, 120 beats/min for 2 min, and 150 beats/min for 6 min). The duration of pacing in each patient is summarized in Table 1. The second angiogram was obtained immediately after discontinuation of pacing. One beat between the 5th and 12th beats after discontinuation of pacing was used for pressure and left ventricular volume analyses. Extrasystolic and post-extrasystolic beats were excluded.

After left ventricular pressure returned to baseline, 10 mg nifedipine was administered sublingually. Ten minutes later baseline pressure recordings were taken, and pacing was repeated at the same rate and duration as before nifedipine. The third angiogram was obtained in the same manner as the second.

Data Analyses

The method of automatic processing of cineangiography has been described elsewhere (Fujita et al. 1981). Briefly, the left ventricular images on cinefilm were transferred to a computer through a flying spot scanner and were stored on magnetic disk. Each digitized image consisted of 128×128 pixels with

Table 1. Patient profiles

Patient no.	Age	Sex	OMI	Coronary anatomy	Baseline LVP/LVEDP (mm Hg)	EDVI (ml/m)	EF (%)	Pacing (min)	Postpacing		Nifedipine and postpacing	
									EDVI (ml/m)	EF (%)	EDVI (ml/m)	EF (%)
1	55	F	–	LAD	182/19	93	47	10	97	38	82	53
2	63	F	–	LAD	154/11	49	68	5	61	54	59	63
3	57	M	–	LMT, LAD	136/16	64	79	3	70	61	64	72
4	70	F	–	LAD	142/8	56	69	7	67	43	56	45
5	71	F	–	RCA	160/10	40	71	7	53	70	52	75
6	44	F	–	LAD	178/16	67	59	10	69	46	76	55
Mean					159/13	62	66	7	70	52	65	61
SD					19/4	18	11	2	15	12	12	12

EDVI, End-diastolic volume index; EF, ejection fraction; LAD, left anterior descending artery; LMT, left main trunk; LVEDP, left ventricular end-diastolic pressure; LVP, left ventricular peak pressure; OMI, old myocardial infarction; RCA, right coronary artery.

gray levels of 256 values. A gradient image was then obtained by spatial differentiation of gray levels. The points with the maximal gradient value were traced to delineate the ventricular boundary.

The left ventricular volumes (V) were calculated by a modification of the formula of Kennedy et al. (1970):

$$V = 0.687\ C^3\ A^2/L + 1.9\ \text{ml}.$$

Where A is the area of the ventricle calculated from the number of pixels surrounded by the left ventricular boundary, L is the longest measured length between the midpoint of the aortic valve and the apex, and C is the linear correction factor for the magnification of a unit of length (1 pixel), which was derived from a comparison with the known area of the filmed 1-cm^2 grid, placed parallel to the tube at the position of the heart.

End-diastole was defined as the timing of the peak of the R wave on the electrocardiogram. Global end-systole was defined as the time when left ventricular volume reaches minimum on the left ventricular volume-time curve, and stroke volume (SV) and ejection fraction (EF) were calculated in the usual fashion. The peak rate of left ventricular filling (LVPF) was obtained from the left ventricular volume-time curve with the use of a digital convolution algorithm developed by Savitzky and coworkers (Sawitzky and Golay 1964).

Unsing an electronic digitizer, we measured left ventricular pressure at approximately 5-ms intervals throughout the period of isovolumic relaxation, defined as the period immediately after maximal negative dP/dt until the time at which pressure had fallen to 5 mmHg above left ventricular end-diastolic pressure. The coordinates of pressure (P) and time (t) were inserted into the equation:

$$P = \mathrm{a} P_0 \exp(-\mathrm{b}t) + \mathrm{c},$$

where P_0 is the pressure at maximal negative dP/dt, exp is exponential, and a, b, c are constants, by the iterative curve-fitting method with use of the algorithm of the steepest descent (Nakamura 1986). The time constant of isovolumic pressure decay (the relaxation time constant) was determined as 1/b (Weiss et al. 1976).

Statistics

To examine the statistical significance of the effect of nifedipine, we tested each parameter in three different stages in the six patients by a two-way analysis of variance, and significant differences were located by the Newman-Keul test. Values for P of less than 0.05 were considered to be significant.

Results

Clinical and Angiographic Characteristics

All patients had a significant stenosis (>75%) in one of the major branches of the coronary artery, and all experienced typical anginal pain during pacing tachycardia. Table 1 summarizes the patient profiles including coronary anatomy, baseline left ventricular pressures, left ventricular end-diastolic volume indices (EDVI), and EF of the beats under three conditions (i.e., baseline, postpacing, and postpacing after administration of nifedipine), and total duration of pacing in each patient. Three sequential left ventricular volume-time curves in a representative case (case 1) are shown in Fig. 1. In the postpacing beat, there was marked reduction in the SV, and with nifedipine the left ventricular volume-time curve returned almost to the preischemic control level.

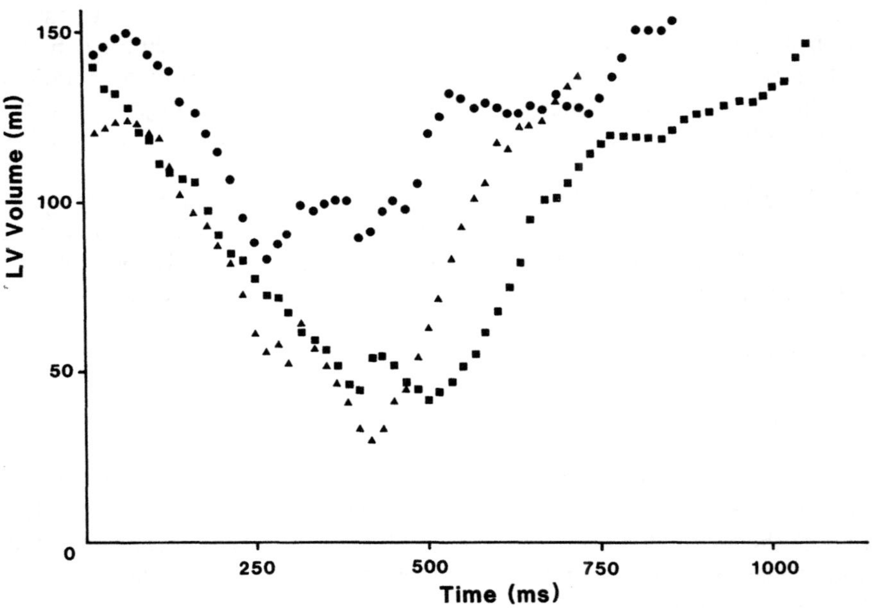

Fig. 1. Three sequential left ventricular volume-time curves obtained by frame-by-frame analysis of left cine ventriculography in a representative case. *Squares* represent data obtained from control left ventriculography, *circles* from postpacing left ventriculography, and *triangles* from postpacing left ventriculography after nifedipine. With pacing-induced ischemia, marked reduction in the stroke volume is seen. After administration of nifedipine, the left ventricular volume-time curve returned almost to the preischemic control curve

Effects of Pacing-Induced Ischemia on Hemodynamics and Ventricular Function

In the postpacing beats, the heart rate did not change significantly (control, 73 ± 12 beats/min versus postpacing, 73 ± 12 beats/min), but the left ventricular peak systolic pressure increased significantly (control, 159 ± 19 mmHg versus postpacing, 180 ± 31 mmHg). There was a substantial increase in left ventricular end-diastolic pressure (LVEDP; control, 13 ± 4 mmHg versus postpacing, 25 ± 4 mmHg; $p < 0.01$). The EF decreased significantly in postpacing beats (control, 65.5 ± 11.1% versus postpacing, 52.0 ± 12.0%; $p < 0.01$). The relaxation time constant increased significantly in postpacing beats (control, 44 ± 10 ms versus postpacing, 62 ± 6 ms; $p < 0.01$), implying impairment of myocardial relaxation with ischemic intervention (Fig. 2).

Both the LVPF and the LVPF normalized for SV (LVPF/SV) tended to increase with ischemic intervention, but not to a statistically significant degree. The LVPF normalized for the end-diastolic volume (LVPF/EDV) did not change after ischemic intervention (LVPF: control, 342 ± 132 ml/s versus postpacing, 361 ± 155 ml/s; LVPF/SV: control, 6.25 ± 3.12 s^{-1} versus postpacing, 7.47 ± 4.68 s^{-1}; LVPF/EDV: control, 4.07 ± 2.27 s^{-1} versus postpac-

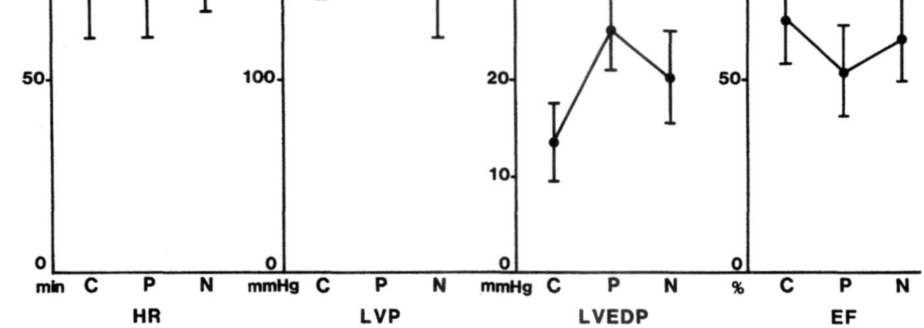

Fig. 2. Effects of pacing-induced ischemia on hemodynamics, ventricular function, and their modification with nifedipine. In the postpacing beat, the peak left ventricular pressure (*LVP*) and the left ventricular end-diastolic pressure (*LVEDP*) increased significantly, but the heart rate did not change. Impairment of ventricular performance is indicated by dercrease in the ejection fraction (*EF*). After the administration of nifedipine (10 mg sublingually), the same duration and the rate of pacing resulted in an increase in the heart rate (*HR*) and changes toward normal in the left ventricular end-diastolic pressure and the ejection fraction. *C*, Control; *P*, postpacing; *N*, postpacing after administration of nifedipine; $^*p < 0.05$; $^{**}p < 0.01$; *NS*, not statistically significant ($n = 6$)

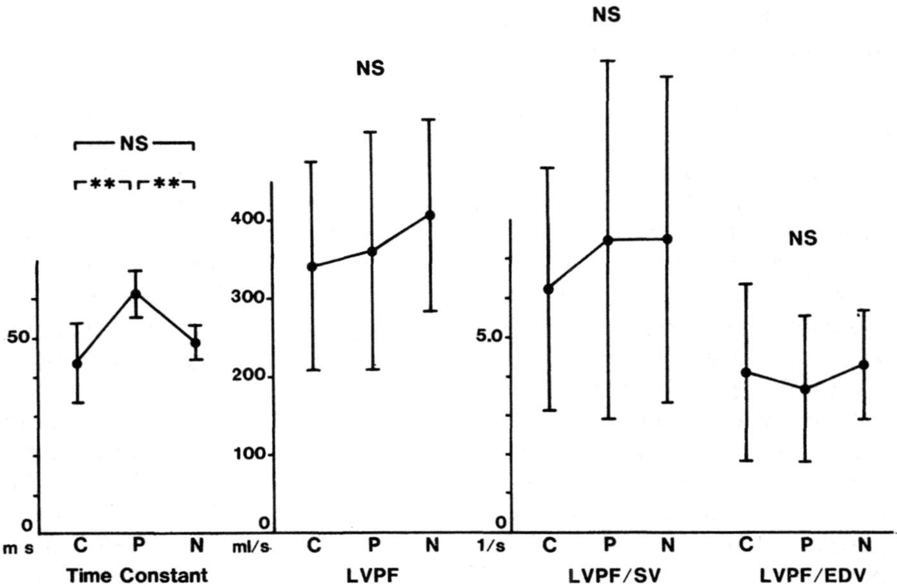

Fig. 3. Effects of pacing-induced ischemia on relaxation time constant, left ventricular filling, and their modification with nifedipine. The relaxation time constant, which increased in postpacing beats, returned toward the preischemic value in postpacing beats after the administration of nifedipine. Although the change did not reach statistical significance, the peak rate of early left ventricular filling (*LVPF*) showed a tendency to increase with nifedipine in the postpacing beat. No significant differences were observed in the LVPF normalized for the stroken volume (*LVPF/SV*) or the LVPF normalized for the end-diastolic volume (*LVPF/EDV*). *C,* Control; *P,* postpacing; *N,* postpacing after administration of nifedipine; $*p<0.05$; $**p<0.01$; *NS,* not statistically significant ($n=6$)

ing, $3.67 \pm 1.84\ s^{-1}$). Thus, pacing-induced ischemia resulted in impairment of left ventricular ejection and relaxation, but it did not appreciably alter global left ventricular filling (Fig. 3).

Modification by Nifedipine of Ischemia-Induced Changes in Hemodynamics and Ventricular Function

The administration of nifedipine resulted in the disappearance or diminution of anginal pain even with the same duration and rates of pacing. After the administration of nifedipine, the same duration and rate of pacing resulted in an increase in the heart rate (86 ± 18 beats/min) and changes towards normal in the LVEDP (20 ± 5 mmHg), EF ($60.5 \pm 11.6\%$), and relaxation time constant (49 ± 4) ms). Both the LVPF and the LVPF/SV tended to increase successively but without statistical significance (LVPF: nifedipine and postpacing, 408 ± 121 ml/s; LVPF/SV: nifedipine and postpacing, 7.52 ± 3.65 sK$-$1).

The LVPF normalized for LVPF/EDV did not change significantly (nifedipine and postpacing, 4.30±1.39 s^{-1}; Figs. 2, 3).

Discussion

The recent interest in diastolic function of the heart has spawned a number of interesting studies dealing with relaxation, early ventricular filling and passive elastic stiffness in a variety of disease conditions (Aroesty et al. 1985; Bonow et al. 1981; Carroll et al. 1983 a, b,; Grossman and Mann 1978; Hammermeister and Warbasse 1974; Hirota 1980; Kumada et al. 1979; McLaurin et al. 1973; Nakamura et al. 1986 a, b; Noble et al. 1969; Paulus et al. 1982; Sasayama et al. 1985; Serizawa et al. 1980; Weisfeldt et al. 1974; Yamagishi et al. 1984). In these studies the effect of ischemia on ventricular filling has been the one of the most important subjects. The LVPF demonstrated by radionuclide angiography in patients with coronary artery disease has been shown to be diminished, and the abnormality of the early ventricular filling has been reported to be independent of left ventricular systolic function and the presence or absence of previous myocardial infarction (Bonow et al. 1981).

However, a recent study by Carroll and coworkers in which left cine ventriculography during exercise was analyzed showed that early left ventricular filling was augmented during exercise in patients with ischemia as well as in patients without ischemia. They showed that the rise in LVPF during exercise was due to a higher filling pressure in patients who developed ischemia (Carroll et al. 1983b). Furthermore, Aroesty and coworkers, who used radionuclide ventriculography during pacing, have also shown that the peak rate of early left ventricular filling was increased during ischemia (Aroesty et al. 1985), but the rise in peak filling rate seen during intermediate levels of pacing tachycardia in patients with ischemic heart disease was blunted or even fell at the highest pacing rates although it stayed at a higher level than the control. They also concluded that the rise in filling rate was induced by the higher left atrial pressure. Thus, both recent studies agree that early left ventricular filling is not impaired but is even augmented during ischemic intervention. They concluded that an increase in left atrial pressure is an important factor causing an increase in the rate of early left ventricular filling during ischemia. The results of global analysis of early left ventricular filling in the present study agree with the findings of these two recent studies. That is, with pacing induced ischemia, despite impairment of ventricular ejection and impairment of relaxation, the rate of early left ventricular filling was not impaired.

The factors that may influence the rate of early left ventricular filling are myocardial systolic shortening, atrioventricular pressure gradient at the time of mitral valve opening, isovolumic relaxation, passive left ventricular compliance, and left ventricular asynchrony (Bahler and Martin 1985; Ishida et al. 1986; Tamiya et al. 1979; Yamagishi et al. 1984). The ischemic process impairs myocardial shortening and relaxation (Grossman and Mann 1978;

Kumada et al. 1979; McLaurin et al. 1973; Paulus et al. 1982; Serizawa et al. 1980; Weisfeldt et al. 1974) and results in asynchrony of left ventricular filling (Kumada et al. 1979; Yamagishi et al. 1984). When a filling pressure or a driving pressure increases, as indicated by an elevation in LVEDP in our study, the peak rate of left ventricular filling should increase substantially. One of the factors that contributes to a blunting of the effect of an increase in a driving pressure on the left ventricular filling rate may be impairment of myocardial distensibility with ischemia. The other factors that we should consider are impairment of left ventricular isovolumic relaxation and accentuated asynchrony in left ventricular filling induced by ischemia. These two factors have been shown previously to affect left ventricular filling (Murakami et al. 1985; Yamagishi et al. 1984).

After the administration of nifedipine, postpacing systolic function and relaxation moved towards their preischemic levels. The beneficial effects of nifedipine on left ventricular response to pacing-induced ischemia in patients with coronary artery disease have been demonstrated by Lorell and coworkers (1981). Their findings regarding the LVEDP, EF, and other indices in 11 of their 17 patients are basically similar to those in the present study. Since they found no changes in left ventricular $+dP/dt$ after nifedipine, a negative inotropic effect was not considered to be the mechanism for the symptomatic and hemodynamic improvement due to nifedipine during ischemia. The mechanism of the beneficial effects of nifedipine in myocardial ischemia has been attributed by Lorell and coworkers, as well as by others, to a decrease in oxygen demand secondary to its unloading effect (Emanuelsson and Holmberg 1983; Nelson et al. 1984; Tiefenbrunn et al. 1983), an increase in oxygen supply due to its vasodilating effect (Henry et al. 1978; Malacoff et al. 1982; Zacca et al. 1982) and to direct protection from ischemic myocardial damage (Henry et al. 1977).

Although it did not reach statistical significance, the LVPF showed a tendency to increase with nifedipine during ischemia. The LVEDP in the postpacing beat after the administration of nifedipine was elevated above the baseline LVEDP in the present study. Therefore, an increase in driving pressure is probably one of the mechanisms of an increase in the three parameters of early left ventricular filling. However, the postpacing LVEDP with nifedipine was lower than that without nifedipine, but the three parameters of the postpacing beat after nifedipine were higher than those without nifedipine. Therefore, an increase in driving pressure alone cannot explain the augmentation with nifedipine of early left ventricular filling. The combined effects of the elevated driving (the left atrial) pressure and improved systolic performance and relaxation may have resulted in improvement in early left ventricular filling with nifedipine in the postpacing beat.

In conclusion, the peak rate of left ventricular filling does not decrease with ischemia despite impairment in systolic performance and isovolumic relaxation due to an increase in left ventricular filling pressure. Nifedipine improves impairment of systolic performance and relaxation caused by ischemia. The early left ventricular filling is facilitated with nifedipine during ischemia by the combined effects of the elevated driving (the left atrial) pressure and improved systolic performance and relaxation.

Acknowledgements: We thank Shigeru Eiho, Ph. D., and Michiyoshi Kuwahara, Ph. D., of Automation Research Laboratory, Kyoto University for help in analyzing the data and Miss S. Hanabuchi for secretarial assistance.

References

Aroesty JM, McKay RG, Heller GV, Royal HD, Als AV, Grossman W (1985) Simultaneous assessment of left ventricular systole and diastolic dysfunction during pacing-induced ischemia. Circulation 71:889

Bahler RC, Martin P (1985) Effects of loading conditions and inotropic state on rapid filling phase of ventricle. Am J Physiol 248:H523

Bonow RD, Bacharach SL, Green MV, Kent KM, Rosing DR, Lipson LC, Leon MB, Epstein ST (1981) Impaired left ventricular diastolic filling in patients with coronary artery disease: assessment with radionuclide angiography. Circulation 64:315

Carroll JD, Hess OM, Hirzel HO, Krayenbuehl HP (1983) Exercise-induced ischemia: the influence of altered relaxation on early diastolic pressures. Circulation 67:521

Carroll JD, Hess OM, Hirzel HO, Krayenbuehl HP (1983b) Dynamics of left ventricular filling at rest and during excercise. Circulation 68:59

Emanuelsson H, Holmberg S (1983) Mechanisms of anginal relief after nifedipine: a hemodynamic and myocardial metabolic study. Circulation 68:124

Fujita M, Sasayama S, Kawai C, Eiho S, Kuwahara M (1981) Automatic processing of cineventriculograms for analysis of regional myocardial function. Circulation 63:1065

Grossman W, Mann JT (1978) Evidence for impaired left ventricular relaxation during acute ischemia in man. Eur J Cardiol 7 [Suppl]:239

Hammermeister KE, Warbasse JR (1974) The rate of change of left ventricular volume in man. II. Diastolic events in health and disease. Circulation 49:739

Henry PD, Shuchleib R, Borda LJ, Roberts R, Williamson JR, Sobel BE (1978) Effects of nifedipine on myocardial perfusion and ischemic injury in dogs. Circ Res 43:372

Henry PD, Shuchleib R, Davis J, Weiss ES, Sobel BE (1977) Myocardial contracture and accumulation of mitochondrial calcium in ischemic rabbit heart. Am J Physiol 233:H677

Hirota Y (1980) A clinical study of left ventricular relaxation. Circulation 69:190

Ishida Y, Meisner JS, Tsujioka K, Gallo JI, Yoran C, Frater RW, Yellin EL (1986) Left ventricular filling dynamics: influence of left ventricular relaxation and left atrial pressure. Circulation 74:187

Kennedy JW, Trenholme SE, Kasser IS (1970) Left ventricular volume and mass from single plane angiogram. A comparison of anteroposterior and right anterior oblique methods. Am Heart J 80:343

Kumade T, Karliner JS, Pouler H, Gallagher KP, Shirato K, Ross J jr (1979) Effects of coronary occlusion on early ventricular diastolic events in conscious dogs. Am J Physiol 237:H542

Lorell BH, Turi Z, Grossman W (1981) Modification of left ventricular response to pacing tachycardia by nifedipine in patients with coronary artery disease. Am J Med 71:667

Lorell BH, Paulus WJ, Grossman W, Wynne J, Cohn PF (1982) Modification of abnormal left ventricular diastolic properties by nifedipine in patients with hypertrophic cardiomyopathy. Circulation 65:499

Malacoff RF, Lorell BH, Mudge GH jr, Holman BL, Idoine J, Bifolck L, Cohn PF (1982) Beneficial effects of nifedipine on regional myocardial blood flow in patients with coronary artery disease. Circulation 65 [Suppl I]:132

McLaurin LP, Rolett EL, Grossman W (1973) Impaired left ventricular relaxation during pacing-induced ischemia. Am J Cardiol 32:751

Murakami T, Hess OM, Krayenbuehl HP (1985) Left ventricular function before and after diltiazem in patients with coronary artery disease. J Am Coll Cardiol 5:723

Nakamura Y, Konishi T, Nonogi H, Sakurai T, Sasayama S, Kawai C (1986) Myocardial relaxation in atrial fibrillation. J Am Coll Cardiol 7:68

Nakamura Y, Wiegner AW, Bing OHL (1986b) Measurement of relaxation in isolated rat ventricular myocardium during hypoxia and reoxygenation. Cadiovasc Res 20:690

Nelson GIC, Slike B, Ahuja RC, Verma SP, Hussain M, Taylor SH (1984) Hemodynamic effects of nifedipine during upright exercise in stable angina pectoris and either normal or severely impaired left ventricular function. Am J Cardiol 53:451

Noble MIN, Milne EN, Goerke RJ, Carlsson E, Domenesch RJ, Sauners KB, Hoffman JIE (1969) Left ventricular filling and diastolic pressure-volume relations in the conscious dog. Circ Res 24:269

Paulus WJ, Serizawa T, Grossman W (1982) Altered left ventricular diastolic properties during pacing-induced ischemia in dogs with coronary stenosis. Potentiations by caffeine. Circ Res 50:218

Sasayama S, Nonogi H, Miyazaki S, Sakurai T, Kawai C, Eiho S, Kuwahara M (1985) Changes in diastolic properties of the regional myocardium during pacing-induced ischemia in human subjects. J Am Coll Cardiol 5:599

Savitzky A, Golay MJE (1964) Smoothing and differentiation of data by simplified least squares procedures. Anal Chem 36:1627

Serizawa T, Carabello BA, Grossmann W (1980) Effect of pacing-induced ischemia on left ventricular diastolic pressure-volume relations in dogs with coronary stenosis. Circ Res 46:430

Tamiya K, Sugawara M, Sakurai Y (1979) Maximum lengthening velocity during isotonic relaxation at preload in canine papillary muscle. Am J Physiol 237:H83

Tiefenbrunn AJ, Sobel BE, Ludbrook PA (1983) Salutary effect of nifedipine in pacing-induced angina: relation to afterload reduction. Cathet Cardiovasc Diagn 9:583

Weisfeldt ML, Armstrong P, Scully HE, Sanders CA, Daggett WM (1974) Incomplete relaxation between beats after myocardial hypoxia and ischemia. J Clin Invest 53:1626

Weiss JL, Frederiksen JW, Weisfeldt ML (1976) Hemodynamic determinants of the time course in canine left ventricular pressure. J Clin Invest 58:751

Yamagishi T, Ozaki M, Kumada T, Ikezono T, Shimizu T, Furutani Y, Yamaoka H, Ogawa H, Matsuzaki M, Matsuda Y, Arima A, Kusukawa R (1984) Asynchronous left ventricular diastolic filling in patients with isolated disease of the left anterior descending coronary artery: assessment with radionuclide ventriculography. Circulation 69:933

Zacca NM, Verani MS, Chahine RA, Miller RR (1982) Effect of nifedipine on exercise-induced left ventricular dysfunction and myocardial hypoperfusion in stable angina. Am J Cardiol 50:689

Atherosclerosis

Effect of Nifedipine on Atherosclerosis in Cholesterol-Fed Rabbits and Watanabe Heritable Hyperlipidemic Rabbits

Y. Ishikawa[1], N. Watanabe[1], N. Miyazaki[1], T. Taniguchi[1], Y. Watanabe[2], and H. Fukuzaki[1]

Introduction

Anticalcifying drugs such as EDTA (Wartman et al. 1967), EHDP (Rosenblum et al. 1975), and thiophene compounds (Chan et al. 1978) have been reported to suppress atherosclerosis in cholesterol-fed rabbits without lowering serum cholesterol levels. Kramsch et al. (1980, 1981) reported that lanthanum, an inorganic calcium antagonist, suppressed atherosclerosis in cholesterol-fed rabbits and monkeys, and Henry and Bentley (1981) demonstrated that nifedipine, a calcium channel blocker, suppressed atherosclerosis in cholesterol-fed rabbits. Thereafter, the calcium channel blockers diltiazem (Ginsburg et al. 1983), verapamil (Rouleau et al. 1983), and nicardipine (Willis et al. 1985) were also reported to suppress atherosclerosis in cholesterol-fed rabbits. However, other investigators have reported that nifedipine (Stender et al. 1984), nicardipine, and diltiazem (Naito et al. 1984) did not suppress atherosclerosis in cholesterol-fed rabbits. In Watanabe heritable hyperlipidemic rabbit (WHHL rabbit; Watanabe 1980), which lacks low-density lipoprotein (LDL) receptors and is a unique model of human familial hypercholesterolemia, Van Niekerk et al. (1984) demonstrated that atherosclerosis was not suppressed by nifedipine.

Therefore, it remains unsolved whether calcium antagonists have antiatherosclerotic effects. We studied the effects of nifedipine on atherosclerosis in both cholesterol-fed rabbits and WHHL rabbits. It is also important to know whether coronary atherosclerosis can be suppressed by nifedipine treatment.

[1] First Department of Internal Medicine, Kobe University School of Medicine, Kobe, Japan
[2] Institute for Experimental Animal, Kobe University School of Medicine, Kobe, Japan

Methods

Cholesterol-Fed Rabbits

Sixteen male Japanese White rabbits aged 3 months were housed individually under a controlled temperature and humidity environment with a 12-h light cycle and were divided into two groups with similar mean values of serum total cholesterol (TC) levels and body weights. One group was fed rabbit chow (ORC-4; Oriental Yeast, Japan) containing 2% cholesterol 120 g/day and administered orally 20 mg nifedipine (a gift from Bayer Yakuhin, Ltd., Japan) twice a day, 7 days a week (nifedipine group). Another group was fed the same diet and administered nifedipine vehicle as a placebo in the same way (placebo group). The experimental period was 3 months. Body weight, serum TC, triglycerides (TG), total calcium, free calcium, GPT, and BUN were measured before treatment and monthly thereafter. Serum TC and TG were analyzed by enzymatic methods, total calcium by the orthocresolphthalein complexone method (Unikit CA; Chugai Pharma, Japan), and free calcium by the ion selective electrode method (SERA-250; Horiba, Japan).

The ultracentrifugation of serum lipoproteins was performed according to the method of Havel et al. (1955) before and after treatment. The serum lipoproteins were divided into four classes: very low density lipoprotein (VLDL; $d<1.006$), intermediate-density lipoprotein (IDL; $1.006<d<1.019$), LDL ($1.019<d<1.063$), and high-density lipoprotein (HDL; $1.063<d<1.210$); levels for TC and TG of each class were measured. Three months after the commencement of treatment, the rabbits were sacrificed with intravenous infusions of pentobarbital sodium solution (100 mg/kg body weight). The whole aorta was removed, cleaned of loosely adhering tissue, and opened longitudinally. Then atherosclerotic lesions were outlined by the xerographic method (Hata et al. 1978) without staining, and the area was measured by planimetry (Planimex 25; Nihon Regulator, Japan). Aortic surface area of atherosclerosis divided by total surface area × 100 was taken as the percentage of atherosclerotic lesion (%AS). The whole aorta was divided into three parts: aortic arch, thoracic aorta, and abdominal aorta. Then the intima-media of each aorta was stripped from the luminal side (Wolinsky and Daly 1970), minced finely, well homogenized, and delipidated with chloroform-methanol 2:1 (vol/vol; Folch et al. 1957).

The aliquot of homogenate was used for the estimation of protein by the method of Lowry et al. (1951). The extract was used for the measurement of TC by enzymatic method (Monotest Cholesterol CHOD-PAP; Boehringer Mannheim Yamanouchi), TG by Fletcher's method (Triglyceride-Test Kit; Wako, Japan). Calcium was extracted from the delipidated tissue by the method of Sparrow and Johnstone (1964) and analyzed by atomic absorption spectrophotometer (Hitachi 207; Hitachi, Japan). Each value was expressed per gram protein. Plasma nifedipine concentrations of four rabbits in the nifedipine group were measured 3 h after high-performance liquid chromatography (Sadanaga et al. 1982) at 5 and 12 weeks. In addition, histological examination was performed to determine the effect of nifedipine on the coronary atherosclerosis. Cardiac ventricles were sliced into three transverse sections. The tissue was fixed with 10% buffered formalin and stained with hematoxylin and eosin. The incidence of atherosclerosis in subepicardial coronary arteries was defined as the number of diseased arteries per total number of arteries.

WHHL Rabbits

The WHHL rabbits were bred in the Institute for Experimental Animals, Kobe University School of Medicine. Fourteen WHHL rabbits aged 3 months (seven males, seven females) were fed standard rabbit chow and divided into two groups with similar mean values of serum TC levels and body weights. Rabbits in the nifedipine group received 20 mg nifedipine twice a day, and rabbits in the placebo group received placebo in the same way. The experimental period was 5 months. Blood samples were drawn from marginal ear veins before and after 1 month, 3 months, and 5 months of treatment. The samples were analyzed as described in the methods for cholesterol-fed rabbits. The ultracentrifugation of serum lipoproteins was also performed at the beginning of treatment and before sacrifice. The WHHL rabbits were sacrificed after 5 months of treatment. The %AS and the tissue lipid and calcium contents were measured in the same way as in the experiment with cholesterol-fed rabbits, and the histological studies of coronary arteries were performed by the same methods as described above.

Statistical Analysis

Comparisons between the two groups were performed by the nonpaired Student's *t* test, and differences between sequential mean values in the same group were evaluated by the paired Student's *t* test. Values were expressed as mean ± standard deviation. The χ^2 test was used for statistical analysis in the histological study.

Results

Cholesterol-Fed Rabbits

Since one of cholesterol-fed rabbits receiving nifedipine died of infection, the numbers of rabbits in the nifedipine group and the placebo group were 7 and 8, respectively. Body weight and serum biochemical measurements are summarized in Table 1. On cholesterol feeding, body weight, GPT, and BUN were increased in both groups, but none of the differences between the two

Table 1. Body weight, GPT, and BUN

		Cholesterol-fed rabbits		WHHL rabbits	
		Before	After	Before	After
Body weight (kg)	P	2.35±0.33	3.05±0.25[a]	2.28±0.32	2.96±0.20[a]
	N	2.36±0.39	2.94±0.36[b]	2.29±0.17	3.01±0.23[a]
GPT (IU/l)	P	20.2±6.5	43.9±27.8[b]	17.5±4.0	28.7±7.9[b]
	N	20.8±7.9	47.0±23.6[b]	16.2±8.2	27.3±9.4
BUN (IU/l)	P	15.9±2.0	30.4± 7.0[a]	16.6±2.4	18.4±3.3
	N	16.5±2.6	31.5±14.5[b]	16.0±4.2	16.0±3.4

P, Placebo group; N, nifidipine group; GPT, glutamate pyruvate transaminase; BUN, blood urea nitrogen. Cholesterol-fed placebo group, $n=8$; cholesterol-fed nifedipine group, $n=7$; WHHL placebo group, $n=6$; WHHL nifedipine group, $n=5$. Differences between nifedipine and placebo groups not statistically significant.

[a] $p<0.01$
[b] $p<0.05$

Table 2. Changes in serum lipid and calcium concentrations

		Before	1 month	2 months	3 months
Cholesterol-fed rabbits					
TC (mg/dl)	P	56.1±11.2	2185±591	2718± 591	2929± 899
	N	55.4±11.0	2187±868	2880±1638	3004±1286
TG (mg/dl)	P	69.8±60.8	172± 80	347±228	557±595
	N	44.9±10.0	219±158	226±194	227±147
Total Ca (mg/dl)	P	14.8±0.7	14.8±0.4	15.0±1.4	15.6±1.3
	N	15.0±0.6	15.2±0.8	14.7±1.4	15.3±0.8
Free Ca (mg/dl)	P	6.5±0.2	6.6±0.3	6.6±0.4	6.7±0.2
	N	6.5±0.2	6.5±0.3	6.3±0.4	6.6±0.2
		Before	1 month	3 months	5 months
WHHL rabbits					
TC (mg/dl)	P	654±193	610± 71	650±58	562± 97
	N	736±146	615±161	650±58	536±134
TG (mg/dl)	P	396±158	277±116	214±51	246± 81
	N	353± 97	302± 51	269±91	267±124
Total Ca (mg/dl)	P	15.0±0.5	15.5±1.1	14.8±1.0	14.7±1.0
	N	14.6±0.4	16.1±0.7	16.1±1.1	15.2±1.1
Free Ca (mg/dl)	P	6.7±0.3	6.7±0.3	6.5±0.6	6.5±0.4
	N	6.4±0.5	6.8±0.2	6.6±0.5	6.5±0.3

P, Placebo group; N, nifedipine group; TC, total cholesterol; TG, triglycerides; Ca, calcium. There were no significant differences between P and N in any measurement. Serum TC and TG increased markedly after cholesterol feeding ($p<0.001$). Total and free calcium levels did not change after drug treatment in cholesterol-fed rabbits or WHHL rabbits.

groups was significant during the experimental period. Plasma nifedipine concentration in the nifedipine group was 1274±561 ng/ml at the 5th week and 1783±747 ng/ml at the 12th week. After 3 months of cholesterol feeding, the serum TC level increased to 2929±899 mg/dl in the placebo group and 3004±1286 mg/dl in the nifedipine group, but no significant differences were found between the two groups (Table 2). Serum TG levels also showed no differences between the groups during the experimental period. Total and free calcium levels in the serum before and after treatment were not different between the groups. Table 3 shows the results of ultracentrifugation of serum lipoproteins performed before and after treatment. VLDL cholesterol was about 1300 mg/dl, IDL cholesterol 800–900 mg/dl, and LDL cholesterol about 600 mg/dl in both groups at the end of the treatment. TG also showed increased levels of VLDL, IDL, and LDL but without differences between groups. Nifedipine had no effect on lipid concentrations in the whole serum or in any fractions in the ultracentrifugation analysis.

Table 3. Ultracentrifugation analysis of serum lipoproteins

		Cholesterol-fed rabbits		WHHL rabbits	
		Before	3 months	Before	3 months
TC (mg/dl)					
Total	P	56.1±11.2	2929± 899	654±193	562± 97
	N	55.4±11.0	3004±1286	736±146	536±134
VLDL	P	2.8±4.1	1346± 581	49±29	25±17
	N	1.4±0.8	1278±1093	43±14	34±19
IDL	P	2.8±3.1	844± 93	47±29	39±26
	N	1.4±0.9	893±236	53±15	40±13
LDL	P	18.4±6.8	602±180	387±223	442± 83
	N	17.2±6.8	614±109	458±119	421±164
HDL	P	19.2±3.9	29.4±12.2	8.8±1.9	5.7±2.2
	N	23.3±7.0	22.1±11.8	6.9±1.1	5.0±1.5
TG (ml/dl)					
Total	P	69.8±60.8	557±595	396±158	246± 81
	N	44.9±10.0	227±147	353± 97	267±124
VLDL	P	18.5±23.1	369±455	56±35	35±23
	N	9.0± 4.4	107± 77	44±15	53±37
IDL	P	8.3±11.9	94±66	31±25	25±14
	N	4.3± 1.7	54±55	26±13	24±15
LDL	P	18.1±11.5	60±40	178±75	160±40
	N	12.5± 3.7	28±12	182±72	165±43
HDL	P	9.7±3.6	5.4±2.8	3.9±1.7	2.0±2.5
	N	8.9±1.5	3.8±2.6	3.7±1.9	2.6±3.0

P, Placebo group; N, nifedipine group; TC, total cholesterol; TG, triglycerides; VLDL, very low-density lipoprotein; IDL, intermediate-density lipoprotein; LDL, low-density lipoprotein; HDL, high-density lipoprotein. Values not significantly different between placebo and nifedipine groups, (nonpaired *t* test).

Table 4. Percentage atherosclerotic lesions of aorta

	Placebo group	Nifedipine group	p
Cholesterol-fed rabbits			
Whole aorta	55.6±22.8	25.9± 7.6	<0.01
Aortic arch	85.9±16.9	68.6±10.7	<0.05
Thoracic aorta	51.1±31.6	8.7± 9.2	<0.005
Abdominal aorta	30.7±24.3	8.6± 4.9	<0.05
WHHL rabbits			
Whole aorta	27.0±11.7	33.4±14.1	NS
Aortic arch	42.2±21.2	45.2±23.0	NS
Thoracic aorta	24.5±11.6	35.5±25.1	NS
Abdominal aorta	15.0± 3.9	19.6± 7.3	NS

NS, Not significantly different between the groups.

The %AS values in the two groups are shown in Table 4 (see also Fig. 1). The %AS of whole aorta averaged 55.6±22.8% in the placebo and 25.9±7.6% in the nifedipine group. There was a significant reduction in atherosclerosis by nifedipine treatment ($p<0.01$). The reduction in atherosclerosis was especially marked in thoracic aorta. The TC content in the whole aorta of the nifedipine group (213±57 mg/g protein) was lower than that of the placebo group (293±130 mg/g protein), although no statistically significant difference was found (Table 5). In thoracic and abdominal aorta, TC contents were significantly lower in the nifedipine group than in the placebo group. The aortic TG contents showed no significant differences between groups. The aortic calcium contents of the two groups were not signifcantly different, but the mean value was about 50% lower in the nifedipine group than in the placebo group. Figure 2 presents microscopic photographs; the atherosclerosis is located primarily in the intramural coronary arteries. The incidence of atherosclerosis in subepicardial arteries was not improved by nifedipine treatment (Table 6).

WHHL Rabbits

Three rabbits, two receiving nifedipine and one receiving placebo, died of infection. There were five WHHL rabbits (three males and two females) in the nifedipine group and six (three males and three females) in the placebo group. Body weight, GPT, and BUN did not vary between groups (Table 1). In our preliminary study, serum nifedipine concentrations elevated to 1447±703 ng/ml ($n=5$) in 6-month-old WHHL rabbits receiving nifedipine twice a day. Serum lipid concentrations decreased with age as reported (Watanabe 1980), but there were no significant differences in TC and TG between nifedipine and placebo groups (Table 2). Total and free calcium levels in the serum were not different between groups (Table 2). Table 3 shows the results of ultracentrifugation of serum lipoproteins. The WHHL rabbits had high levels of

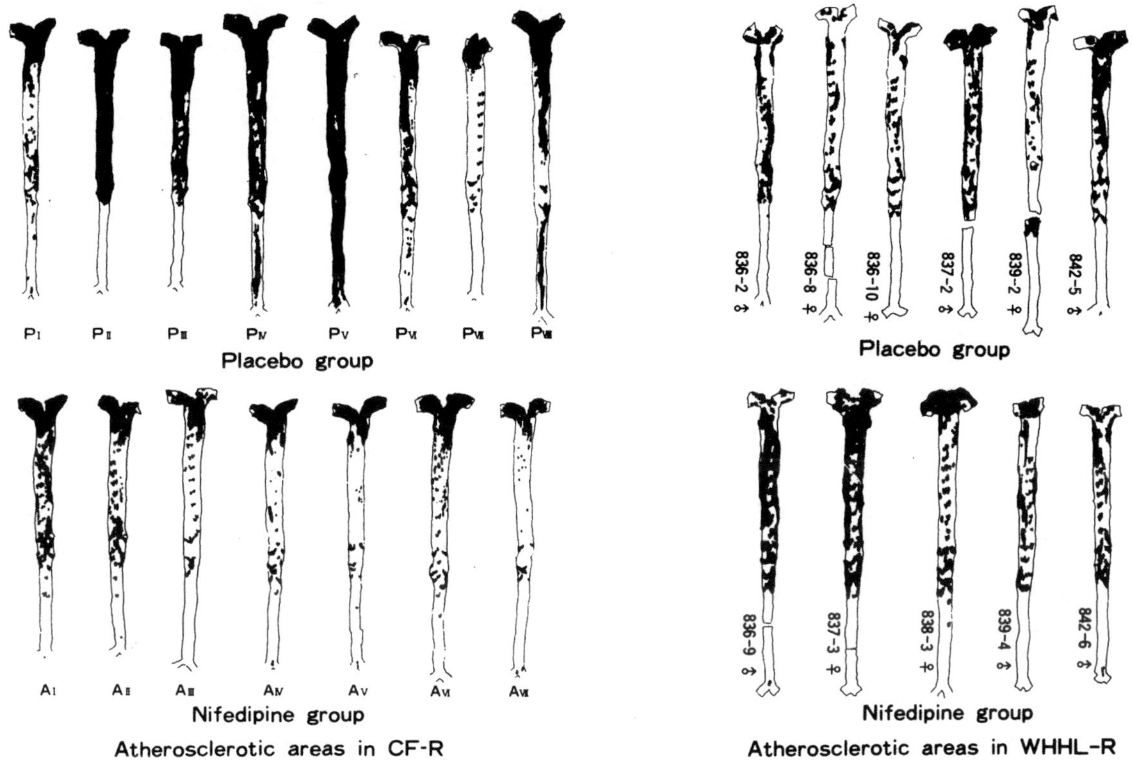

Fig. 1. Atherosclerotic areas by xerographic method. After sacrifice of the rabbits, the whole aortas were removed, cleaned of loosely adhering tissue, and opened longitudinally. Atherosclerotic lesions were then outlined by the xerographic method. The nifedipine group showed markedly smaller atherosclerotic lesions than the placebo group in cholesterol-fed rabbits (*CF-R*), whereas the two groups showed about the same degree of atherosclerosis in Watanabe heritable hyperlipidemic rabbits (*WHHL-R*)

Table 5. Tissue lipid and calcium contents

		Cholesterol-fed rabbits				WHHL rabbits			
		Whole aorta	Aortic arch	Thoracic aorta	Abdominal aorta	Whole aorta	Aortic arch	Thoracic aorta	Abdominal aorta
Cholesterol	P	293±130	519±248	176±115 ⎤ *	179±104 ⎤ *	243± 60	337± 71	186± 69	151±46
(mg/g protein)	N	213± 57	471±179	51± 37 ⎦	71± 19 ⎦	303±133	306±170	209±134	194±83
Triglycerides	P	12±5.5	12±5	11±10	16±11	87±79	84±111	52±34	139±11
(mg/g protein)	N	9.1±3.6	10±4	8.1±5.9	8.3±3.8	30± 7	35±8.6	27±20	33±22
Calcium	P	3.9±4.4	5.8±8.1	2.2±1.1	2.7±0.7	6.4±2.7	7.4±3.6	5.5±3.1	6.1±2.1
(mg/g protein)	N	2.0±1.3	2.1±1.5	1.1±0.2	3.0±2.6	10.5±6.6	14.4±8.0	5.1±4.4	9.8±8.9

P, Placebo group; N, nifedipine group.

* $p < 0.05$ (nonpaired student's t test)

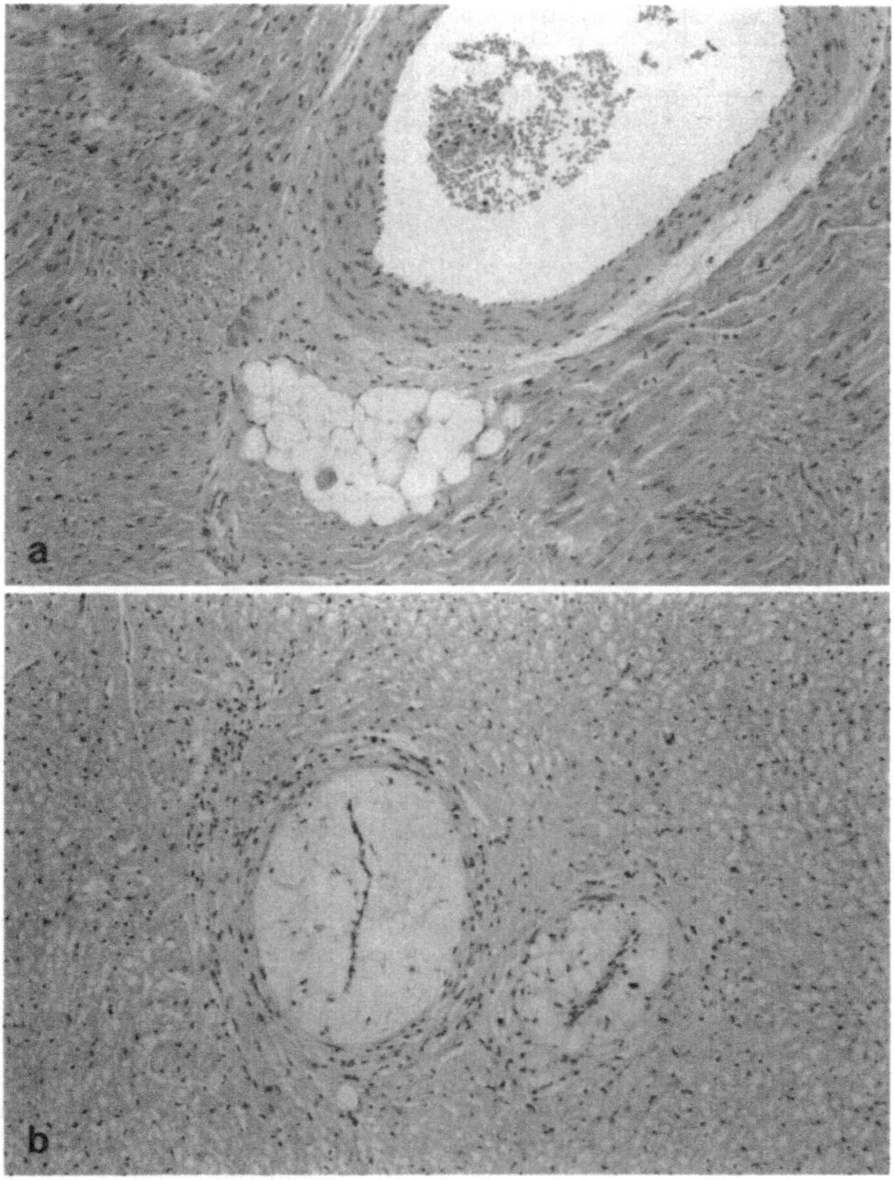

Fig. 2a, b. Micrograph of coronary arteries from cholesterol-fed rabbit treated with nifedipine. **a** Subepicardial coronary vessel (hematoxylin and eosin). **b** Intramural coronary vessels showing proliferation of lipid laden cells (hematoxylin and eosin)

Table 6. Incidence of atherosclerosis in coronary arteries

	Cholesterol-fed rabbits	WHHL rabbits
Nifedipine group	7/99 (7.1%)	2/65 (3.1%)
Placebo group	8/93 (8.6%)	7/75 (9.3%)

VLDL, IDL, and LDL as compared with normal Japanese White rabbits, but there were no significant differences in any fractions between groups.

The extent of atherosclerosis in both groups are shown in Fig. 1 and Table 4. There was no significant difference in %AS of the whole aorta between the groups. Each part of the aorta showed the same result. Tissue lipid and calcium contents showed no differences in the whole aorta or in any parts of the aorta. As shown in Table 6, there was no difference in the incidence of coronary atherosclerosis between groups.

Discussion

In our experiments, nifedipine effectively suppressed atherosclerosis in cholesterol-fed rabbits but not in WHHL rabbits. In cholesterol-fed rabbits, the nifedipine group had significantly lower %AS values than the placebo group in the whole aorta ($p<0.01$). Each part of the aorta in the nifedipine group also had a significantly lower %AS value than in the placebo group (aortic arch, $p<0.05$; thoracic aorta, $p<0.005$; abdominal aorta, $p<0.05$), and the reduction in atherosclerosis was especially marked in the thoracic aorta. TC and calcium contents of thoracic aorta in the nifedipine group were also significantly lower than in the placebo group. On the other hand, in WHHL rabbits no significant differences were obtained in %AS, tissue TC, or calcium content. Our results in WHHL rabbits are consistent with those of Van Niekerk et al. (1984).

Numerous mechanisms by which calcium antagonists may suppress atherosclerosis have been proposed. Henry and Bentley (1981) suggested that calcium antagonists may protect against cell necrosis, which could be an initial event in atherosclerosis, and suppress a chain of processes thereafter. Another possibility is that calcium antagonists interfere with the key enzymes of lipid metabolism such as cholesterol ester hydrolase and cholesterol synthetase. Recently, Etingin and Hajja (1985) reported that nifedipine increased lysosomal and cytoplasmic cholesterol ester hydrolytic activity in cultured rabbit arterial smooth-muscle cells. In our study, the serum lipid levels were not different between nifedipine and placebo groups either in the total contents or in any fractions in ultracentrifugation. Therefore, cholesterol catabolism in the arterial wall may be enhanced by nifedipine treatment.

Other investigators have suggested many other possibilities, such as the suppression of the proliferation and migration of smooth-muscle cells (Nakao et al. 1983) and the promotion of PGI_2 synthesis in endothelial cells and smooth-muscle cells (Terashita et al. 1984). The lowering of blood pressure has also been considered to be antiatherogenic. However, Blumlein et al. (1984) showed that while verapamil suppressed atherosclerosis in cholesterol-fed rabbits, blood pressure in the experimental group was not different from that in the control group. Henry and Bentley (1981) reported that the decrease in blood pressure by nifedipine was only transient, lasting 2 h. Therfore, the antihypertensive effect of nifedipine does not seem to play an important role in preventing atherosclerosis. Since the process of atherosclerosis is multifactorial, the effect of calcium antagonists is probably not by a single mechanism.

To explain our discrepant results in cholesterol-fed rabbits and WHHL rabbits, we should emphasize the possibility that nifedipine affects LDL receptor activity. Recently, Stein et al. (1985) reported that verapamil enhanced LDL receptor-mediated uptake and degradation of LDL in endothelial and smooth-muscle cells, probably by increasing receptor numbers. By promoting LDL Cholesterol catabolism, calcium antagonists may prevent the accumulation of cholesterol ester. This may be one of the beneficial effects of nifedipine in suppressing atherosclerosis. We should also take into consideration that the nature of cells alters as the atherosclerosis progresses. According to morphological observation (Yoshida et al. 1983), smooth-muscle cells that migrated into the intima altered their phenotype from contractile to synthetic type when rabbits were fed a high-cholesterol diet for 1 week. Thus, the smooth-muscle cells may change in character as the atherosclerosis advances. Since WHHL rabbits have been exposed to hyperlipidemic serum from birth, the nature of the smooth-cells may already have been changed functionally from the beginning of the experiment, even if this was not shown microscopically. This would lead to ineffectiveness of nifedipine in suppressing atherosclerosis in WHHL rabbits. Naito et al. (1984) reported that calcium antagonists were not effective in the atherosclerosis of cholesterol-fed rabbits. However, they started drug treatment after 2 weeks of high-cholesterol feeding. The differences between our results and theirs may be due to this. Therefore, we can conclude that nifedipine seems to suppress atherosclerosis in the earlier stages.

In coronary arteries, subepicardial vessels showed less severe lesions compared to intramural vessels. The treatment of nifedipine had no effect on the incidence of coronary atherosclerosis in either type of vessel.

We studied the effects of nifedipine on atherosclerosis in cholesterol-fed and WHHL rabbits, and the two groups of rabbits showed different responses. These results suggest that the effect of nifedipine may be mediated by LDL receptors, or that the early exposure to hyperlipidemic serum from birth in WHHL rabbits may have an affect on cell functions.

Acknowledgements: We thank Dr. Ryozo Okamoto, Dr. Shinji Takano, Dr. Manabu Tsukitani, and Dr. Junichi Mukodani for their helpful discussions, and Ms. Shoko Iwai for manuscript preparation.

References

Blumlein SL, Sievers R, Kidd P, Parmley WW (1984) Mechanism of protection from atherosclerosis by verapamil in the cholesterol-fed rabbit. Am J Cardiol 54:884–889

Chan CT, Wells H, Kramsch DM (1978) Suppression of calcific fibrous-fatty plaque formation in rabbits by agents not affecting elevated serum cholesterol levels. The effect of thiophene compounds. Circ Res 43:115–125

Etingin OR, Hajjar DP (1985) Nifedipine increases cholesteryl ester hydrolytic activity in lipid-laden rabbit arterial smooth muscle cells. A possible mechanism for its antiatherogenic effect. J Clin Invest 75:1554–1558

Folch J, Lees M, Sloane Stanley GH (1957) A simple method for the isolation and purification of total lipids from animal tissues. J Biol Chem 226:497–509

Ginsburg R, Davis K, Bristow MR et al. (1983) Calcium antagonists suppress atherogenesis in aorta but not the intramural coronary arteries of cholesterol-fed rabbits. Lab Invest 49:154–158

Hata Y, Shigematsu H, Tsushima M, Aihara K (1978) A xerographic method for the quantitative assessment of atherosclerotic lesions. Atherosclerosis 29:251–258

Havel RJ, Eder HA, Bragdon JH (1955) The distribution and chemical composition of ultracentrifugally separated lipoproteins in human serum. J Clin Invest 34:1345–1353

Henry PD, Bentley KI (1981) Suppression of atherogenesis in cholesterol-fed rabbit treated with nifedipine. J Clin Invest 68:1366–1369

Kramsch DM, Aspen AJ, Apstein CS (1980) Suppression of experimental atherosclerosis by the Ca -antagonist lanthanum. J Clin Invest 65:967–981

Kramsch DM, Aspen AJ, Rozler LJ (1981) Atherosclerosis: prevention by agents not affecting abnormal levels of blood lipids. Science 213:1511–1512

Lowry OH, Rosebrough NJ, Farr AL, Randall RJ (1951) Protein measurement with the Folin phenol reagent. J Biol Chem 193:265–275

Naito M, Kuzuya F, Asai K, Shibata K, Yoshimine N (1984) Ineffectiveness of Ca -anagonists nicardipine and diltiazem on experimental atherosclerosis in cholesterol-fed rabbits. Atherosclerosis 51:343–344

Nakao J, Ito H, Ooyama T, Chang WC, Murota S (1983) Calcium dependency of aortic smooth muscle cell migration induced by 12-L-hydroxy-5, 8, 10, 14-eicosatetraenoic acid. Effect of A23187, nicardipine and trifluoperazine. Atherosclerosis 46:309–319

Rosenblum IY, Flora L, Eisenstein R (1975) The effect of disodium ethane-1-hydroxy-1, 1-diphosphonate (EHDP) on a rabbit model of athero-arteriosclerosis. Atherosclerosis 22:411–424

Rouleau JL, Parmley WW, Stevens J et al (1983) Verapamil suppresses atherosclerosis in cholesterol-fed rabbits. J Am Coll Cardiol 1:1453–1460

Sadanaga T, Hikida K, Tameto K, Matsushima Y, Ohkura Y (1982) Determination of nifedipine in plasma by high-performance liquid chromatography. Chem Pharm Bull (Tokyo) 30:3807–3809

Sparrow MP, Johnstone BM (1964) A rapid micro-method for extraction of Ca and Mg from tissue. Biochim Biophys Acta 90:425–426

Stein O, Leitersdorf E, Stein Y (1985) Verapamil enhances receptor-mediated endocytosis of low density lipoproteins by aortic cells in culture. Arteriosclerosis 5:35–44

Stender S, Stender I, Nordestgaard B, Kjeldsen K (1984) No effect of nifedipine on atherogenesis in cholesterol-fed rabbits. Arteriosclerosis 4:389–394

Terashita K, Orimo H, Nakamura T, Ooshima J, Harasawa M (1984) Calcium metabolism and arteriosclerosis, I: the effect of Ca-antagonist on the release of PGI_2 from cultured rat aortic smooth muscle cells. J Jpn Atheroscler Soc 12:851–856 (English abstr)

Van Niekerk JLM, Hendriks T, De Boer HHM, Van't Laar A (1984) Does nifedipine suppress atherogenesis in WHHL rabbits? Atherosclerosis 52:91–98

Wartmann A, Lampe TL, McCann DS, Boyle AJ (1967) Plaque reversal with Mg EDTA in experimental atherosclerosis: elastin and collagen metabolism. J Atheroscler Res 7:331–341

Watanabe Y (1980) Serial inbreeding of rabbits with hereditary hyperlipidema (WHHL-rabbit). Incidence and development of atherosclerosis and xanthoma. Atherosclerosis 36:261–268

Willis AL, Nagel B, Churchill V et al. (1985) Antiatherosclerotic effects of nicardipine and nifedipine in cholesterol-fed rabbits. Arteriosclerosis 5:250–255

Wolinsky H, Daly MM (1970) A method for the isolation of intima-media samples from arteries. Proc Soc Exp Biol Med 135:364–368

Yoshida Y, Mitsumata M, Ooneda G, Takatama M (1983) Growth of smooth muscle cells in aortic atherosclerotic plaques of rabbits. J Jpn Atheroscler Soc 11:1165–1172 (English abstr)

Natural History of Coronary Artery Disease: The Effects of Ca^{2+} Channel Blockade and Antiplatelet Agent on Progression or Regression of Coronary Atherosclerosis

Y. Yabe[1]

Introduction

Myocardial infarction (MI) is the major cause of death in the natural history of coronary artery disease. The initial attack of MI and reinfarction are closely related to the progression of coronary arteriosclerosis. In other words, coronary artery disease is a progressive disease, and it is essential to understand clinically the rate and nature of progression. On the other hand, however, one sometimes also observes the regression of a stenosis on a coronary angiogram. Nevertheless, the actual mechanisms are not fully understood. This chapter discusses the natural history of coronary artery diseases and the influence of long-term administration of a calcium antagonist, based on the findings of coronary angiography.

Subjects and Methods

The subjects of this study were 252 patients with stable-effort angina who had received coronary angiography more than twice, with a follow-up interval ranging from 6 to 60 months (average, 12.4 months). Of these 252 cases, 96 (group 1) received medical treatment and 156 (group 2) received surgical treatment (coronary artery bypass). Mean age was 54.5 years in group 1 and 54.1 in group 2.

Groups 1 and 2 were divided into subgroups A, B, and C depending on the drug used (see Table 1). Group B received long-term administration of either trapidil (300 mg/day) or dipyridamole (75 mg/day) plus aspirin (300 mg/day). Group C received long-term administration of the calcium antagonist nifedipine (40 mg/day). To group A was administered neither an antiplatelet agent nor a calcium antagonist; this group served as control. Coronary angiogram was conducted according to the Sones method, and cases with positive ergonovine test and spontaneous spasm were excluded. Angiography was conducted under intra-aortic sinus administration of 5 mg isosorbide dinitrate

[1] Cardiovascular Diagnostic Laboratory Center, Toho University School of Medicine, Tokyo, Japan

Table 1. Number of subjects in groups and subgroups

Subgroups	Groups 1. Medical treatment	Groups 2. Surgical treatment	Total
A. Control	38	46	84
B. Antiplatelet agent			
Trapidil 300 mg/day	37 [25	80 [30	117
Dipyridamole 75 mg + aspirin 300 mg/day	12	50	
C. Ca antagonist			
Nifedipine 40 mg/day	21	30	51
Total	96	156	252

Table 2. Classification schema for progression/regression in coronary atherosclerosis. (From Kramer et al. [2])

Progression
(1) From less than 100% to 100%
(2) From less than 70% to 90% or more
(3) From less than 30% to greater than 50%
(4) A 20 % or more increase of obstruction in any vessel narrowed by 50% or more

Regression
(1) Any change from total obstruction to less than total obstruction
(2) Any reduction in lumen diameter obstruction of 20% or more

in all cases. Percent stenosis evaluation was conducted both according to the methods of the American Heart Association classification and by autoanalysis of the percent diameter stenosis on real-time basis [1]. In group 2 we studied the nongrafted native coronary artery. Statistical analysis was conducted using the nonpaired t test and the χ^2 test. The schema of Kramer et al. [2] was used for the classification of disease progression and regression (Table 2). Those cases which could not be classified as showing either progression or regression were classified as nonprogression.

Results

Age of Patients and Progression

Group A, which received no antiprogressive treatment, showed progression rates of 63% and 67% for those aged under 40 and over 60, respectively (Fig. 1). These rates are high regardless of age. The figures for groups B and C were 0% and 38%, and 0% and 50%, respectively. In comparison to group A,

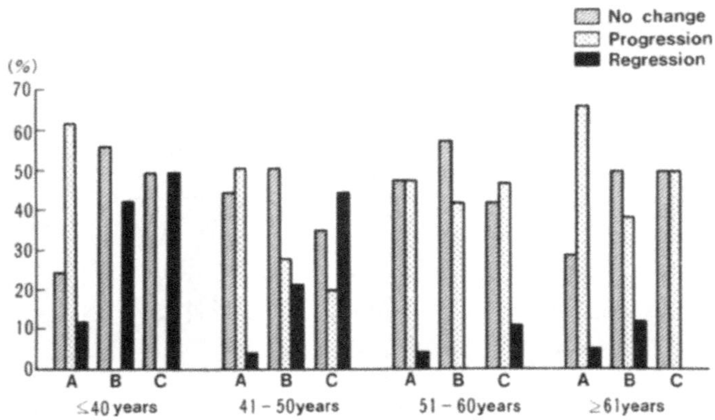

Fig. 1. Relationship between change in disease and age of patient in groups A, B, and C

groups B and C thus clearly showed lower rates of progression. There was no statistically significant difference between group B and group C, but a significant difference did exist between group A and groups B and C ($p<0.05$). Regarding cases of nonprogression, both B and C groups exceeded 50% for the age groups under 40 and over 60, in contrast to rates of 25% and 28% in group A.

Follow-up Interval and Progression

In the case of a short follow-up period of less than 12 months, the progression rate was 46% in group A and 31% in groups B and C (Fig. 2). However, in the case of a follow-up interval of 1–2 years, progression rates were 67%, 60%, and 72% in groups A, B, and C, respectively. The progression rate was high regardless of treatment method. This indicates the proportional relationship between extension of the follow-up interval and progression of the disease.

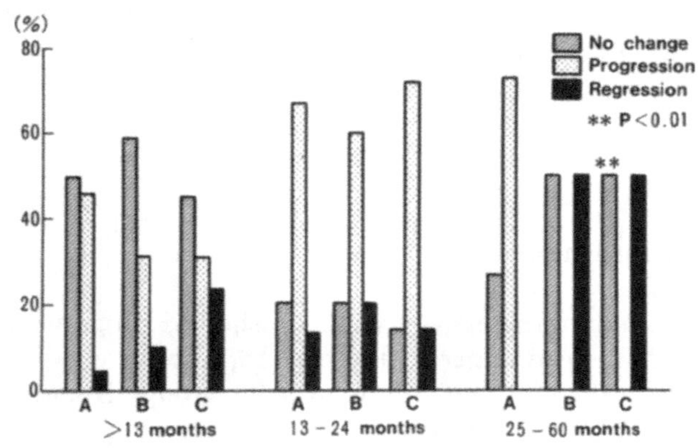

Fig. 2. Relationship between change in disease and interval of follow-up in groups A, B, and C

On the other hand, in the case of a follow-up interval of more than 2 years, a different tendency was observed. In group A, the progression rate hight of 73% and the increase in the rate were proportional to the extension of the follow-up interval. However, in groups B and C progression was not observed (perhaps due to the small number of cases), and nonprogression and regression showed high rates. There was a significant difference between group A and groups B and C in terms of nonprogression, progression, and regression ($p<0.01$).

Number of Affected Vessels and Progression

Regarding single-vessel disease, progression of the disease in the angina-related vessel, especially the initial lesion, was 67% in group A, 51% in group B, and 50% in group C (Fig. 3). Also, new lesions on other vessels were observed. Between 22% and 33% showed progression to two-vessel disease, and 11%–18% showed progression to three-vessel disease. In the case of multiple-vessel disease (that with more than two vessels affected), a difference was observed between group A and groups B and C. Regarding the rate of progression, 10%–50% of group A patients (average, 43%) showed progression in angina-related vessels. In contrast, excluding four cases of progression to two-vessel disease in group B, there was no progression to multiple-vessel disease. Statistically, a significant difference was observed between group A and groups B and C regarding three-vessel disease ($p<0.05$).

Progression in Group with Medical Treatment

Among 612 vessels of coronary arteries, progression was observed in 70 vessels. The frequency of progression in terms of the number of vessels affected was 11.4% (Fig. 4). Kramer's type 1 progression (from high-grade lesion to

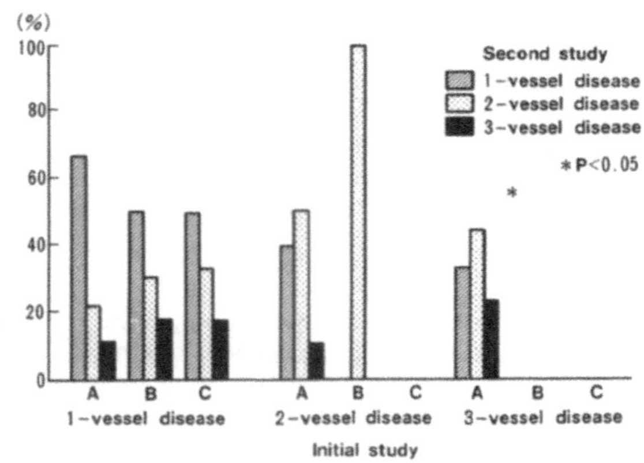

Fig. 3. Relationship between number of affected vessels at initial examination and that of vessels with progression at second examination in groups A, B, and C

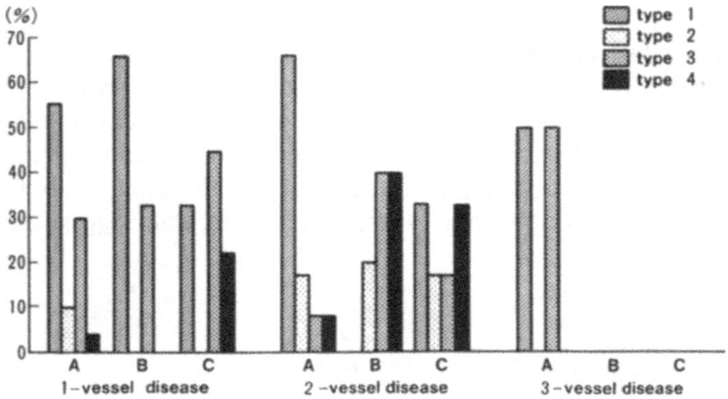

Fig. 4. Percentage of cases showing progression, by number of affected vessels and type of progression, in subgroups A, B, and C of group 1

total occlusion) was highest in group A regardless of the number of affected vessels. Type 1 progression of one-, two-, and three-vessel disease was 56%, 67%, and 50%, respectively (average, 58%). This indicates a high incidence of progression to MI in this group. However, in groups B and C the rates of type 1 progression of one-vessel disease were 67% and 33%, respectively. The incidence was thus high for group B. In the case of multiple-vessel disease, the rate of type 1 progression was not as high, but that of types 3 and 4 were increased. For groups B and C the figures were: type 1, 31% and 33%; type 2, 86% and 5%, type 3, 38% and 29%; and type 4, 23% and 33%. The number of cases showing moderate progression was greater. The number of cases which progressed to MI were decreased.

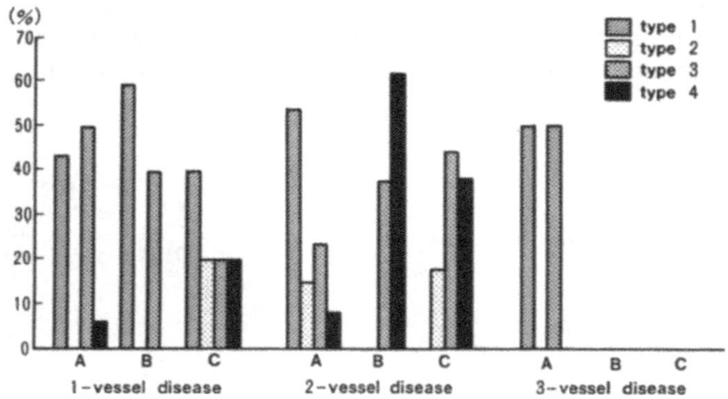

Fig. 5. Percentage of cases showing progression, by number of affected vessels and type of progression, in subgroups A, B, and C of group 2

Progression in Group with Surgical Treatment

Among 625 total vessels of coronary arteries, 71 showed progression, and the rate of progression was 11.3% (Fig. 5). There was no difference between groups 1 and 2 as to the rate of progression, but the type of progression was different. Types 1 and 3 were observed in 49% and 40%, respectively, in group A. Progression rates of types 1, 3, and 4 in groups B and C were 31% and 38%, 35% and 31%, and 35% and 31%, respectively. The distribution was thus rather similar in groups B and C. The fact that type 1 progression of non-grafted native coronary artery was 30% in group B and 21% in group C is important for the long-term evaluation of surgical results.

Type of Treatment and Natural History of Disease

The comparison of natural history during a follow-up interval of 12–12.7 months (average, 12.4 months; Fig. 6 shows rates of nonprogression, progression, and regression in group A of 44%, 55%, and 5%; in group B of 54%, 33%, and 13%; and in group C of 44%, 35%, and 21%. It should be noted that the regression rate was highest in group C. There was no statistically significant difference between groups B and C, but a significant difference was observed between group A and groups B and C in terms of nonprogression, progression, and regression ($p<0.01$).

Type of Treatment and Global Left Ventricular Function at First and Second Examinations (Table 3)

Hemodynamic indices obtained at initial and second cardiac catheterization were compared in group 1 (Table 3). In group A, there was a tendency to decreasing cardiac index (CI), left ventricular dP/dt/P, and a tendency to

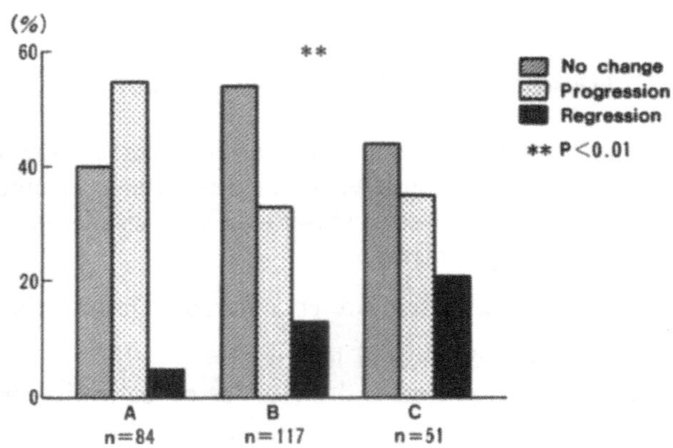

Fig. 6. Natural history of disease in groups A, B, and C

Table 3. Left ventricular performance at first and second examinations

Hemodynamic parameter	Examination	Control ($n=38$)	Trapidil treatment ($n=24$)	Nifedipine treatment ($n=21$)
Cardiac index	1st	3.22±0.79	2.60±0.22	2.55±0.60
	2nd	3.06±0.74	3.20±0.24	3.17±0.50
End-diastolic pressure	1st	14.8±7.1	14.0±1.1	14.5±2.1
(mm Hg)	2nd	15.9±6.3	13.8±1.2	12.0±1.5
End-diastolic volume	1st	93.8±39.5	98.0±7.0	101.5±5.0
index	2nd	95.6±39.7	80.5±6.8	90.1±3.0
Ejection fraction (%)	1st	55.8±17.4	63.2±5.8	50.2±2.3
	2nd	54.3±21.0	61.1±5.9	55.5±5.4
dP/dt/P	1st	41.6±11.8	34.0±3.5	31.0±2.5
(s^{-1})	2nd	39.7±9.9	37.0±3.6	33.5±3.1
Stroke work index	1st	77.9±25.6	104.1±5.7	85.0±5.0
	2nd	77.3±40.2	100.6±5.9	90.0±9.0
Systolic pressure index	1st	252.1±93.8	315.2±10.5	300.5±5.0
	2nd	22.55±79.1	214.3±12.4	312.5±7.4
N dP/dt	1st	2481±735	2413±110	2300±150
	2nd	7769±101	2252±66	2100±70

increasing LV end-diastolic pressure (LVEDP), and LV end-diastolic volume index (LVEDVI), although significant differences were not observed. In group B (24 cases of long-term trapidil administration) an increase in CI ($p<0.02$) and LV dP/dt/P ($p<0.02$) against baseline was observed. At the same time, LVEDP significantly decreased ($p<0.05$). In group C, significant increases in CI, LV dP/dt/P, and ejection fraction ($p<0.05$) and a significant decrease in LVEDP ($p<0.02$) were observed. In comparison to group A, global LV function was improved in group C.

Discussion

Characteristics of Progression in Control Group

As regards organ specificity of arteriosclerosis, the natural history of coronary arteriosclerosis (stable-effort angina) was evaluated in terms of progression, nonprogression, and regression. Evaluation was carried out by consecutive coronary angiography.

The following factors are considered to induce the progression of diseases:

(a) size and location of lesion,
(b) sustained period and incidence of ischemic condition,
(c) coexistence of spasm and abnormal tonus of coronary artery,

(d) development of collateral circulation,
(e) age of patient,
(f) coronary risk factor,
(g) systemic hemodynamic conditions,
(h) progression of platelet aggregation, and
(i) calcium ion deposition on arterial wall.

In group A there was no significant difference among age groups; the progression rate was over 50% regardless of age. Among patients aged below 40 years, 63% exhibited progression. This indicates that, in the case of coronary arteries, the rate of progression does not necessarily correlate with age.

In regard to the length of follow-up interval, the progression rate was highest (73%) when the follow-up interval exceeded 2 years. As has been reported by other researchers, it seems that a sustained period of ischemia and the frequency of anginal attacks affect the progression of the disease. Significant progression was observed in 46% of 54 cases which had the shorter follow-up interval of less than 2 years. This fact is also important in evaluating the patients with angina.

In terms of the number of affected vessels, 67% of cases with single-vessel disease, showed progression of disease at the initial site. This figure is rather high, and among those with progression, 56% could be classified as type 1. Together with the fact that other researchers have reported a high mortality rate among patients with restenosed single-vessel disease, the above findings indicate that even in single-vessel disease it is possible for the disease to progress to fatal MI. Thus it is considered essential for the clinical management of angina to make adequate evaluation of the disease and to select optimum timing for the performance of percutaneous TCA.

To summarize the various factors such as age, sex, and follow-up interval of group A, the average rate of progression among 38 cases (34 men, 4 women; average age, 51.6 years) was 55%. This figure is similar to the rate of 71% reported by Rösch et al. [4] with an average follow-up interval of 29 months and that of 68.5% reported by Kimbiris et al. [5], with an average follow-up interval of 26.2 months. Although rather short, this interval is enough to predict the natural history of coronary artery disease. We cannot neglect the importance of early reexamination of patients by coronary angiography. Among the total of 1237 coronary artery vessels in our study, progression was observed in 141 arteries, for a progression rate of 11.4%. This figure corresponds well with the results of Rösch et al. [4] (12.6%) and those of Nobuyoshi et al. [6] (10.6%).

Arteriosclerosis is said to be a progressive disease, and it is questioned whether there may be a natural regression of progressed arteriosclerosis of the coronary artery. We actually encountered such regression – as shown by coronary angiography – in 5% of cases in group A (control). The characteristics of this regression are shown in the change from Kramer type 1 (total occlusion) to nonocclusive disease. We rarely observed regression from significant stenosis to nonsignificant stenosis. This fact suggests that in the control group regression was caused mainly by the thrombolysis and resultant recanalization of the infarction-related coronary artery.

Characteristics and Mechanism of Progression or Regression in Drug-Treated Groups

As the cause of the progression of atherosclerosis, the role of platelet viscosity and aggregation as the hemostatic mechanism has gained attention in recent years, in addition to such factors as those of atherosclerotic plaque and damaged endothelial cells. It has also been reported that arachidonic acid is released from membrane phospholipids by the activation of platelets which cause the synthesis of thromboxane A_2 (TXA_2), followed by the enhancement of platelet aggregation and hence vasospasm, which is the important factor of ischemia, and leading to myocardial ischemia, unstable angina, and finally MI and sudden death [7]. Aspirin, sulfinpyrazone, dipyridamole (Persantine), and trapidil are well-known antiplatelet agents. In vivo and in vitro effects of these agents against atherosclerosis are well established, however, reports on the clinical study of coronary artery are rather limited.

Chesebro et al. [8] conducted long-term administration of 75 mg dipyridamole and 325 mg aspirin 7 h after the operation and compared the potency of the graft against that in a placebo group. Of the 478 grafts in the drug-treated group, 11% showed occlusion, against 23% of 468 grafts in the placebo group; this difference is significant. They reported that the combined use of dipyridamole and aspirin contributed not only to the short-term but also to the long-term potency of grafts, and that the mechanism may be the delay of progression of atherosclerosis by the suppression of platelet activity. However, their study was limited to the graft artery after the operation, and they did not refer to the influence on nongrafted arteries. Trapidil is also said to have potent coronary dilatation and antihyperlipidemia activities. At the same time, it is said to inhibit TXA_2 synthesis, to have antiplatelet activity similar to that of aspirin, and to promote PGI_2 synthesis. However, reports on the effect of long-term administration of this drug on coronary atherosclerosis are limited [9].

The role of calcium ion in the genesis and progression of arteriosclerosis has gained attention in recent years. In the case of smooth muscle of artery, calcium ion overload is considered to be an important factor of atherogenesis which leads to necrosis or calcification of vessels. Research on the effect of calcium antagonists on atherogenesis is still at an experimental stage, and studies on the coronary artery are scarce.

Kramsch et al. [10] administered the inorganic calcium ion antagonist, lanthanum chloride, to cholesterol-fed rabbits and demonstrated the suppression of experimental atherosclerosis after 8 weeks treatment.

Henry [11] created atherosclerosis in rabbit by 2% cholesterol and administered orally 40 mg nifedipine per day for 8 weeks. In the placebo group, the density of cholesterol and calcium in aortic tissue, which occupied $40 \pm 5\%$ of the endothelium of the aortic lesion stained by Sudan IV, was 47 ± 5 mg/g protein and 297 ± 18μg/g protein. In the nifedipine group, area of lesion, cholesterol, and calcium had decreased significantly to 17 ± 3%, 29 ± 2 mg/g protein, and 202 ± 14 μg/g protein on average, respectively. Based on these findings, it was reported that the dihydropyridine agent nifedipine can suppress morphological and biochemical changes of atherosclerosis without improving hypercholersterolemia. That is, the calcium antagonist suppresses necrosis of the vessel wall, and nifedipine suppresses cellular turnover or atherogenesis. Fleckenstein and Witzleben [12] administered 50–150 mg nifedipine per day for 5 months to diabetic rats and spontaneously hypertensive rats and observed that the agent normalized blood pressure and prevented abnormal deposition of calcium ion on the arterial wall. They proposed that appropriate treatment by a calcium antagonist could suppress calcium overload on the arterial wall and have a protective effect on experimental vessel damage and may thus play a role in preventing the progression of arteriosclerosis.

On the other hand, Ginsberg et al. [13] administered diltiazem and reported that it suppressed aortic sclerosis, but they could not observe the effect on the coronary artery. There are several other reports which deny the effect of the calcium antagonist. In Japan, Naito et al. [14] studied the effect of diltiazem on cultured smooth muscle of aortic tunica media.

Other than the above-mentioned effect, the calcium antagonist suppresses vasospasm, has hypotensive effect, and affects platelet function, prostanoid metabolism, and lipid metabolism. This agent always provides stimulus to the clinical cardioangiology area. This agent contains complex factors which cannot be explained simply by the specific activity on smooth muscle or after load reduction. One must conclude that several factors act synergistically or cooperatively.

It has already been stated that coronary spasm and enhancement of platelet aggregation as well as coronary arteriosclerosis are closely related to coronary circulation disorder. Maseri et al. [15], considering that these features are related to the pathogenesis of coronary circulation disorder, proposed the viscious circle of coronary artery disorder (coronary arteriosclerosis, spasm, hemodynamic changes around the lesion, endothelial cell damage, enhancement of platelet aggregation, release of the vasoconstrictive substance TXA_2) to be the mechanism of the progression of coronary artery disease. It has been shown that nifedipine can stop this cycle by its clear antispasm effect, morphological and biochemical suppression of atherogenesis, and antiplatelet activity. Thus it can prevent the progression of disease and occurrence of MI. Ross et al. [16] emphasized the interrelationship of endothelial cell damage, platelets, and macrophages on atherogenesis. They stated that damage to the endothelium is the key event, and that elucidation of the mechanism of this event may lead to the prevention and diagnosis of atherosclerosis and the application of nonsurgical coronary revascularization procedures such as PTCA. Nifedipine and antiplatelet agents may act favorably on the above-mentioned relationship.

However, there have been few clinical studies on the effect of nifedipine on atherogenesis. In particular, there has been no report on the natural history of sclerotic coronary artery disease when a clinically optimum dose is administered for a long period of time.

In order to assess the agreement between theoretical and clinical features, the present author administered daily doses of 300 mg trapidil or 75 mg dipyridamole plus 300 mg aspirin as antiplatelet agent and 40 mg nifedipine as calcium antagonist for more than 6 months. Subjects were patients with stable-effort angina caused by organic coronary artery disease. Administration of drugs was initiated immediately after the initial coronary angiography and terminated at the second angiogram. The results were compared to those among controls. There were no statistical differences in regard to the background factors of age, sex, follow-up interval, etc. between groups B and C, treated by the antiplatelet agent or calcium antagonist to prevent disease progression. Compared to group A, the progression rate of elderly patients (those aged over 60 years) in groups B and C was significantly lower than that of those in group A, at 38% and 50%. Also, there was no case of pogression in patients under 40 years of age in groups B and C. Of note is the fact that the rate of nonprogression was high in groups B and C.

Regarding the relationship to follow-up interval, there was no significant difference observed with a follow-up period of under 2 years. However, when the interval exceeded 25 months, there was no case of progression in groups B and C, and significant differences were observed against group A. This indicates the favorable effect of long-term administration of these agents. Concerning the relationship to the number of affected vessels, the number of cases which progressed either from initial one-vessel to multiple-vessel or from initial multiple-vessel to vessels in other arteries was small, although the population itself was small in comparison to that of group A. With regard to the type of progression, 67% of patients in group B and 33% in group C with single-vessel disease showed type 1 progression. The progression rate was lowest in group C. However, in reference to patients with two- or three-vessel disease, the rate of type 1 progression was as low as 0%–33%, and the other cases belonged to types 3 and 4. There was a tendency to low MI incidence in groups B and C. This suggests that both agents act favorably in terms of speed and degree of disease progression. However, as regards the difference between group A and groups B and C in multiple-vessel disease, we should take into account not only the specific activity and synergistic effects of these vessels but also the influence of collateral circulation, increase of flow rate by the dilatation of coronary arteries, and the avoidance of pump failure after load reduction.

The natural history of groups B and C was compared with that of group A at an average follow-up interval of 12.4 months. Nonprogression, progression, and regression rates in group B were 54%, 33%, and 13%, respectively. In comparison to group A, nonprogression was significantly high ($p<0.01$) and progression significantly low ($p<0.01$). With regard to group C, nonprogression was significantly low at 44% ($p<0.01$), and the regression rate of 21% was the highest among the three groups. There was no significant difference between groups B and C. From the above it can be observed that trapidil, dipyridamole plus aspirin as antiplatelet agent, and the calcium antagonist nifedipine, when consistently administered for a long period of time, can prevent the progression of coronary artery disease. The results also indicate that both agents contribute to regression of the disease.

We have already noted the importance of coronary arteriosclerosis and spasm in ischemic heart disease. Vasospasm is active at the organic lesion. Marzilli et al. [17] specified coronary spasm as the mechanism of coronary sclerosis. It has also been indicated that repeated coronary spasm at the organic lesion can promote the progression of atherosclerosis. The pathogenesis of coronary spasm, however, is not yet known. The natural history and long-term results of vasospastic angina such as atypical angina are thought to have favorable prognosis, and there are several aspects which do not agree with the above-mentioned hypothesis. Further detailed study is required to determine whether coronary spasm is the mechanism of progression.

With regard to the regression of coronary artery disease, the mechanism is considered to be thrombolysis in group A because the majority of cases in this group belong to type 1. The regression rate is highest in group C, and more than 40% of those showing regression can be classified as type 2 regression. In addition to thrombolysis, suppression of coronary spasm by these agents, the influence of lipid metabolism, calcium on arterial wall, and the synergistic effects of these factors are considered to be the mechanism of regression in this group.

Our data show only the two-dimensional luminal changes of coronary arteries by coronary arteriography. The problem in our data is the lack of direct proof of regression, as direct observation of histological changes of the tunica media or changes at the cellular level is not possible. It would be premature to conclude that the phenomena observed are caused by specific and synergistic effects of these agents. Nevertheless, in our study the regression rate was significantly higher in groups B and C in comparison to control ($p<0.01$) especially in patients of younger age. The relationship between time of regression and change in morphology, thrombolysis, the influence on long-term results, and the duration of administration are the important factors which require further investigation.

Conclusions

The natural history of medically or surgically treated coronary artery disease shows progression at 1-year follow-up to be as high of 55% regardless of age, if no measures are taken to prevent progression. The degree of progression corresponds to the length of follow-up interval. As regards type of progression, the rate of progression to total occlusion is the highest (53%) in group A. This factor contributed to the high mortality rate (18.7%), reinfarction rate (24.4%), and unfavorable long-term results attack but also the prevention of progression should be considered in the treatment of angina.

The group receiving long-term administration of either antiplatelet agent (trapidil 300 mg/day or dipyridamole 75 mg plus aspirin 300 mg/day) or calcium antagonist (nifedipine 40 mg/day) exhibited higher rates of nonprogression than control. The progression rates were 33% and 35%, which were significantly lower than that of the control group. This tendency is more prominent in multiple-vessel disease. Regarding type of progression, the percentage of type 1 was low, and remaining cases were distributed among types 3 or 4. It was indicated that the degree of progression could be improved. If the administration of antiplatelet agent and the calcium antagonist nifedipine extends to more than 2 years, these drugs are considered to contribute to the prevention of disease progression. Also, it was indicated that nifedipine might influence the regression of the disease. Suppression of platelet aggregation, influence on prostanoid metabolism, improvement of lipid metabolism, suppression of vessel damage and coronary spasm, and the synergistic or cooperative effect of these factors are considered to cause the regression. At the same time, influence on LV function and effect of coronary dilatation should be taken into account.

For angina, selection of a more appropriate palliative treatment method, such as antianginal drug, PTCA, or coronary artery bypass graft, of course, is essential. But treatment should include not only the suppression of angina attack but also a specific program for the prevention of progression.

References

1. Yamashita T, Yabe Y (1985) Study on automated analysis of stenotic rate and effect of PTCA procedure on real time basis. Med Biol Eng Comput 23 [Suppl]:256
2. Kramer JR, Matsuda Y, Mullingan JC et al (1981) Progression of coronary atherosclerosis. Circulation 63:519
3. Suzuki S, Inoue Y, Taira A et al (1984) Natural history of myocardial infarction in terms of coronary arteriographical findings (in Japanese). Kokyu To Junkan 32:65
4. Rösch J, Rahimtoola SH (1977) Progression of angiographically determined coronary stenosis. In: Rahimtoola SH (ed) Coronary bypass surgery. Davis, Philadelphia
5. Kombiris D, Lavine D, Van Den Brock H et al (1974) Devolutionary pattern of coronary atherosclerosis in patients with angina pectoris. Coronary angiographic studies. Am J Cardiol 33:7
6. Nobuyoshi M, Nosaka H, Ito K (1980) A study on progression of coronary artery disease by serial coronary arteriography (in Japanese). Sinzo 12:496
7. Maseri A, Chierchia S, L'Abbate A (1980) Pathogenetic mechanisms underlying the clinical events associated with atherosclerotic heart disease. Circulation 62 [Suppl 5]:3–13
8. Chesebro JH, Fuster V, Elverback LR (1984) Effect of dipyridamole and aspirin on late vein graft potency after coronary bypass operation. N Engl J Med 310:209
9. Onishi H, Ito R (1979) Experimental study on effect of trapidil on synthesis of thromboxane A2, platelet aggregation, vasoconstriction and ischemic heart disease. Atherosclerosis 7:407
10. Kramsch DM, Aspen AJ, Apstein CS (1980) Suppression of experimental atherosclerosis by the CAV-antagonist lanthanum. Possible role of calcium in atherogenesis. J Clin Invest 65:967

11. Henry PD (1982) Nifedipine suppresses atherogenesis in cholesterol-fed rabbit. In: Kaltenback M, Neufeld HN (eds) Proceeding of 5th International Adalat Symposium, Berlin 1982. Excerpta Medica, Amsterdam, pp 55–61
12. Fleckenstein A, Witzleben FM (1982) Vascular calcium overload — a pathogenetic factor in arteriosclerosis and its neutralization by calcium antagonists. In: Kaltenback M, Neufeld HN (eds) Proceeding of 5th International Adalat Symposium, Berlin 1982. Excerpta Medica, Amsterdam, pp 36–52
13. Ginsburg R, Davis K, Schroeder JS (1983) Calcium antagonists suppress atherogenesis in aorta but not in the intramural coronary arteries of cholesterol-fed rabbits. Lab Invest 49:154
14. Naito M, Asai K, Shibata K (1984) The effect of Ca^{2+} antagonists on bovine aortic smooth muscle cells in culture. Atherosclerosis 12:845
15. Maseri A, L'Abbate A, Chierchia S et al (1981) Ischemic heart disease in the 1980s — the role of spasms in angina pectoris and infarction, indications for future research and therapy. Pract Cardiol 7:29
16. Ross R, Faggiotto A, Bowen-Pope D (1984) The role of endothelial injury and platelet and macrophage interaction in atherosclerosis. Circulation 70 [Suppl III]:III–77
17. Marzilli M, Goldstein S, Maseri A et al (1980) Some clinical considerations regarding the relation of coronary vasospasm to coronary atherosclerosis. A hypothetical pathogenesis. Am J Cardiol 45:882

Effect of Nifedipine on DNA Synthesis and Cytosolic Free Calcium Concentration Stimulated by Growth Factors: A Study Using Cultured Rat Aortic Smooth-Muscle Cells

Y. Ouchi[1], J. Hirosumi[1], M. Watanabe[1], J. Kusunoki[1], and H. Orimo[1]

Introduction

Recently, calcium antagonists such as nifedipine and lanthanum have been reported by many investigators to have an antiatherogenic action (Rosenblum et al. 1975; Kramsch et al. 1980; Henry and Bentley 1981), and it has been suggested that calcium ion may play an important role in the development of atherosclerosis. However, the mechanism has not been fully understood. On the other hand, some kinds of growth factors, such as platelet-derived growth factor (PDGF) and epidermal growth factor (EGF), have been known to increase calcium ion concentration in the target cells with or without accompanying the activation of C kinase (Berridge and Irvine 1984; Hesketh et al. 1985), and the increase in cytosolic calcium concentration may trigger the DNA synthesis of the target cells (Campbell 1983). A recent major observation in atheromatous plaque has been the migration and proliferation of smooth-muscle cells (SMCs), and some kinds of growth factors are suggested to be at least in part responsible for this phenomenon (Ross et al. 1974; Ross and Glomset 1976; Ross 1986). We therefore studied the effects of growth factors on DNA synthesis and cytosolic free calcium concentration and also the effect of nifedipine on the action of growth factors, using aortic SMCs derived from rats.

Materials and Methods

Cell Culture: SMCs were aseptically isolated from aortic media of male Wistar rats 5–6 weeks old using the explant method developed by Ross (1971). Primary culture was performed in M199 (Nissui, Japan) containing 20% fetal calf serum (FCS; Gibco, USA) in plastic dishes under 95% air and 5% CO_2 at 37 °C. SMCs became confluent after around 2 weeks, and the cells were detached from dishes with trypsin (0.125%) and ethylenediamine tetraacetic acid (EDTA; 0.005%). The cells were transferred to an other plastic dish, and cul-

[1] Department of Geriatrics, University of Tokyo, Tokyo, Japan

ture was continued in minimal essential medium (MEM, Nissui, Japan) containing 10% FCS. SMCs at the tenth passage were used in this study.

Measurement of Cytosolic Free Calcium Concentration: SMCs were inoculated onto round glass coverslips of 13.5 mm diameter and 0.12 mm thickness. When the cells became confluent, MEM containing 0.1% FCS was substituted for the medium to arrest the cells. After 24 h, SMCs were labeled with quin 2/AM. MEM containing 0.1% FCS was discarded, and 0.5 ml MEM containing 30 μM quin 2/AM (Wako, Japan) was added. After incubation for 20 min, the medium was diluted four times with MEM, and the cells were incubated for an additional 30 min. The glass coverslips were washed and transferred into quartz cuvette containing 1.3 ml simplified medium (145 mM NaCl, 5 mM KCl, 1 mM Na_2HPO_4, 1 mM $CaCl_2$, 0.5 mM $MgSO_4$, 5 mM glucose, and 10 mM HEPES; pH 7.4). The cuvettes were placed in spectrophotometer (Hitachi 650-10S), and fluorescence was measured with an excitation wave length of 339 nm using 4 nm for a slit and an excitation wave length of 492 nm using 10 nm for a slit. Cytosolic free calcium concentration was calculated using the method developed by Tsien et al. (Tsien et al. 1982; Capponi et al. 1985). The effects of PDGF (Collaborative Research, USA), EGF (Collaborative Research, USA), and somatomedin C (Sm-C; Fujisawa Pharmaceutical, Japan) with or without nifedipine (Bayer, FRG) or verapamil (Eisai, Japan) on the cytosolic free calcium concentration were studied by the serial measurements of fluorescence for 10 min.

Measurement of DNA Synthesis: SMCs were inoculated onto 96 multiwell plastic dishes (0.32 cm^2/well) and were cultured until confluency. After the growth of the cells was arrested by the substitution of MEM containing 0.1% FCS for the previous medium, [^{3}H]thymidine (New England Nuclear, USA) of 1 μCi/ml was added with or without growth factors and with or without calcium antagonists. Incubation was terminated by discarding the medium containing [^{3}H]thymidine and washing twice with simplified medium. Cells were incubated in 0.1 ml 5% trichloroacetic acid for 20 min and then lysed with 50 μl NaOH (0.5 N). The cell lysate was neutralized with the same amount of 0.5 N of HCl and was transferred to a counting vial, and 1 ml Pico-Fluor (Packard Instruments, USA) was added. Radioactivity of the mixture was measured with a liquid scintilation counter (Aloka LSC 700, Japan) and was considered to be the amount of DNA synthesis in SMCs.

Results

Effect of Growth Factors on Cytosolic Free Calcium Concentration in SMC: Cytosolic free calcium concentration before treatments by growth factors was 178 ± 18 nM ($n = 15$). As shown in the inset of Fig. 1, PDGF (1 U/ml) evoked a transient and significant increase in cytosolic calcium concentration in SMCs. Cytosolic free calcium concentration became maximal after 3 min and

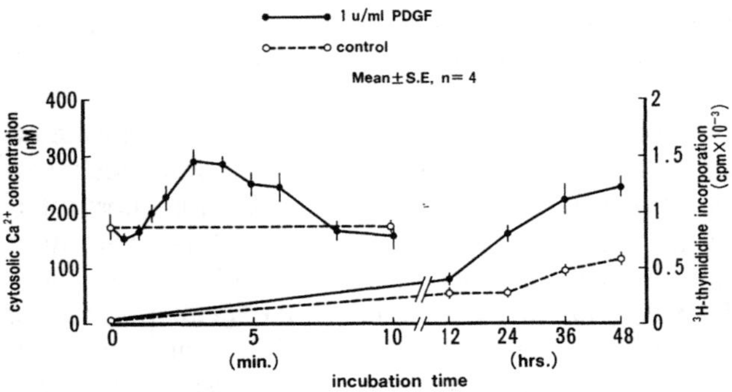

Fig. 1. Time course change in [^{3}H]thymidine incorporation and cytosolic free calcium concentration *(inset)* in SMCs treated with 1 U/ml PDGF

then gradually fell to the baseline level. The administration of the same amount of phosphate buffered saline (PBS) for vehicle did not alter the cytosolic free calcium concentration. EGF (100 ng/ml) also evoked the significant increase in cytosolic free calcium concentration, as shown in the inset of Fig. 2. The magnitude of the increment in cytosolic free calcium concentration was greater in response to EGF than to PDGF. However, as shown in the inset of Fig. 3, Sm-C (100 ng/ml) did not affect the cytosolic free calcium concentration in SMCs.

Effect of Growth Factors on DNA Synthesis in SMC: Serial measurements of [^{3}H]thymidine incorporation into SMCs showed that DNA synthesis gradually increased with time and reached a plateau level after 36 h incubation (controls in Figs. 1, 2, 3). Like PDGF and EGF (Figs. 1, 2), Sm-C significantly enhanced DNA synthesis, although it did not affect the cytosolic free calcium concentration (Fig. 3).

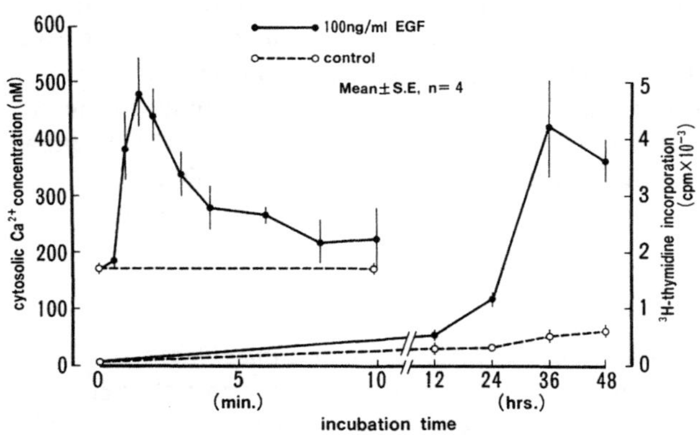

Fig. 2. Time course change in [^{3}H]thymidine incorporation and cytosolic free calcium concentration *(inset)* in SMCs treated with 100 ng/ml EGF

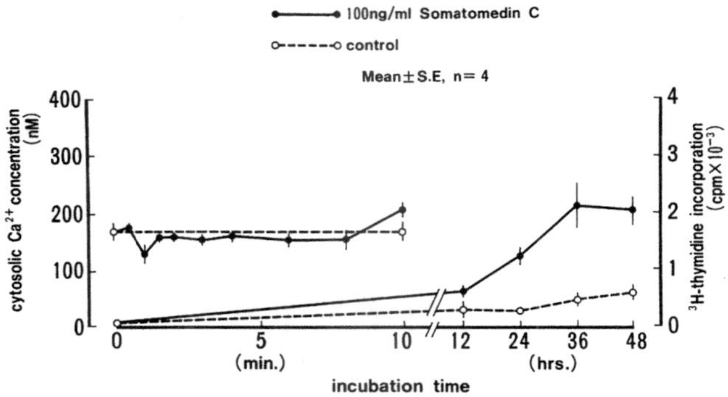

Fig. 3. Time course change in [^{3}H]thymidine incorporation and cytosolic free calcium concentration *(inset)* in SMCs treated with somatomedin C (100 ng/ml)

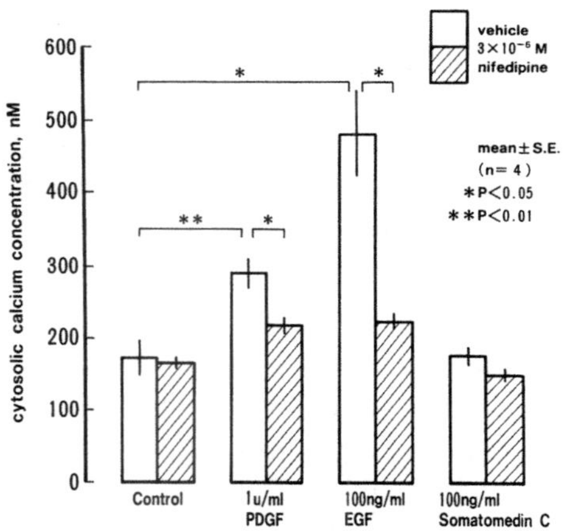

Fig. 4. Effects of nifedipine on peak values of cytosolic free calcium concentration in SMCs without treatments (control) and in SMCs treated with 1 U/ml PDGF, 100 ng/ml EGF, and 100 ng/ml somatomedin C

Effect of Nifedipine on Cytosolic Free Calcium Concentration in SMC: Figure 4 shows the effects of the concomitant administration of nifedipine (3×10^{-6} *M*) on cytosolic free calcium concentration in SMC. As shown in the left column, cytosolic free calcium concentration was not altered by nifedipine alone, while the increase in cytosolic free calcium concentration evoked by PDGF and EGF was significantly inhibited. Sm-C again did not affect the cytosolic free calcium concentration, as shown in the right column. Nifedipine, administered together with Sm-C, also had no effect on cytosolic free calcium concentration in SMC.

Effect of Nifedipine on DNA Synthesis in SMC: As shown in Fig. 5, PDGF, EGF, and Sm-C significantly enhanced DNA synthesis. Nifedipine (3×10^{-6} *M*) significantly inhibited the enhancement of DNA synthesis in response to EGF but did not inhibit the enhancement evoked by PDGF and Sm-C.

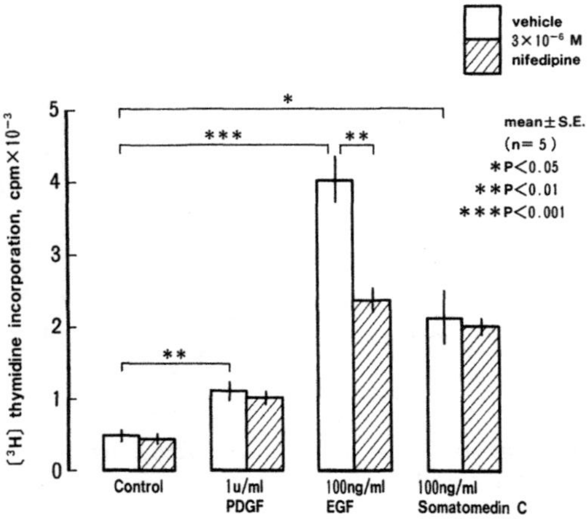

Fig. 5. Effects of nifedipine on [^{3}H]thymidine incorporation after 36-h treatment with 1 U/ml PDGF, 100 ng/ml EGF, and 100 ng/ml somatomedin C. Control cells were incubated with vehicle (PBS) not containing growth factors (control)

Effects of Verapamil on Cytosolic Free Calcium Concentration and DNA Synthesis in SMC: The left panel of Fig. 6 shows the effects of verapamil on the increase in cytosolic free calcium concentration evoked by EGF: verapamil inhibited the increase in cytosolic free calcium concentration in a dose-dependent manner. The right panel of Fig.6 shows the effect of verapamil on the enhancement of DNA synthesis evoked by EGF: verapamil also inhibited DNA synthesis evoked by EGF.

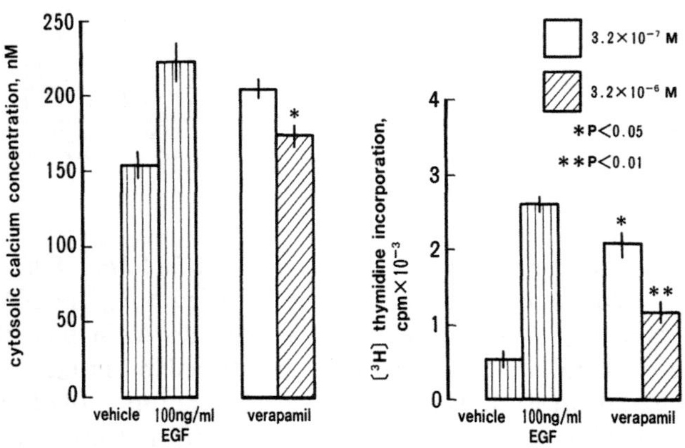

Fig. 6. Effects of verapamil on peak values of cytosolic free calcium concentration *(left panel)* and [^{3}H]thymidine incorporation *(right panel)* after 36-h treatment with 100 ng/ml; * $p<0.05$, ** $p<0.01$ vs. 100 ng/ml EGF

Discussion

Proliferation of SMCs in the arterial intima has been reported to be one of the major phenomena in atherogenesis since Ross et al. (Ross and Glomset 1976; Ross 1986) proposed the response-to-injury hypothesis. They suggest that PDGF has some role in the proliferation of vascular SMCs in the progression of atherosclerosis; however, the mechanism has not been fully understood. Furthermore, EGF is also suggested to have some role in the proliferation of vascular SMCs (Berk et al. 1985).

In this study we have demonstrated that EGF evokes the enhancement of DNA synthesis in cultured SMCs, and that the enhancement is associated with an increase in cytosolic free calcium concentration. Cytosolic calcium ion has been shown to play an important role in some cellular functions, such as muscle contraction, secretion of biological products, cell division, cell migration, and gene expression (Campbell 1983). Our results indicate that cytosolic calcium ion may also be involved in the proliferation of vascular SMCs in response to EGF. This was supported by the observation that the pretreatment of the cultured SMCs with the calcium antagonist nifedipine inhibited the enhancement of DNA synthesis evoked by EGF.

The effect of nifedipine on PDGF-induced DNA synthesis was somewhat different from that observed in the case of EGF. Although PDGF-evoked enhancement of DNA synthesis was associated with an increase in cytosolic free calcium concentration in SMCs, and the increase was well inhibited by nifedipine, nifedipine had only minimal inhibitory action on DNA synthesis. To explain the discrepancy, two possibilities must be considered. First, PDGF is known to activate phospholipase C and to generate inositol (1, 4, 5)-trisphosphate (IP_3) in the cell membrane, and the IP_3 mobilizes Ca^{2+} into cells (Berridge and Irvine 1984). Diacylglycerol (DG) is also generated, and protein kinase C is activated. Thus, both IP_3 and DG are reported to be responsible for the promotion of DNA synthesis in response to PDGF. On the other hand, EGF is reported to evoke the influx of Ca^{2+} into cells without accompanying the generation of IP_3 and activation of C kinase in 3T3 fibroblasts (Hesketh et al. 1985). Hence, the minimal inhibitory effect of nifedipine on PDGF-induced DNA synthesis may be explained by the hypothesis that only one pathway, either IP_3 or DG, is necessary for the promotion of DNA synthesis in vascular SMCs. In other words, even if nifedipine inhibits the mobilization of Ca^{2+} into cytosol, the generation of DG followed by activation of proteine kinase C may be enough to promote DNA synthesis. The second possibility is that PDGF promotes DNA synthesis by the mechanism independent of cytosolic calcium. Unfortunately, we have no evidence to determine the actual mechanism.

In contrast to PGDF and EGF, Sm-C enhanced DNA synthesis without any effect on the cytosolic free calcium concentration. Moreover, nifedipine had no effects on the enhancement of DNA synthesis evoked by Sm-C. Accordingly, Sm-C may have a mechanism independent of cytosolic calcium to stimulate DNA synthesis.

In the present study, verapamil, another calcium antagonist, was also found to inhibit the increase in cytosolic free calcium concentration and DNA synthesis evoked by EGF. This result suggests that the effects of nifedipine on cytosolic free calcium concentration and DNA synthesis are not mediated by pharmacological action other than the calcium-antagonistic action but are mediated by the calcium-antagonistic action.

Although the mechanisms of antiatherogenic action of calcium antagonists have not been fully elucidated, several possiblilities have been suggested. Nakao et al. (1983) showed calcium antagonists inhibited the migration of arterial SMCs using modified Boyden chamber. Stein et al. (1985) and Etingin and Hajjar (1985) showed that calcium antagonists could interfere with low-density lipoprotein metabolism or cholesterol metabolism in arterial SMCs. The data presented in this study indicate the possibility that calcium antagonists inhibit the growth factor mediated proliferation of arterial SMCs, and this may be one mechanism to explain the antiatherogenic action of calcium antagonists.

In conclusion, both PDGF and EGF increased DNA synthesis and cytosolic free calcium concentration in aortic SMCs, but only EGF-induced DNA synthesis was inhibited by nifedipine. EGF-induced increase in DNA synthesis was dependent on the increase in the cytosolic free calcium concentration, while another mechanism may be involved in PDGF-induced increase in DNA synthesis. On the other hand, Sm-C increased DNA synthesis independent of cytosolic free calcium concentration. These result suggest that the cellular mechanism of the proliferation of SMCs may differ among growth factors, and that the inhibitory action of nifedipine on EGF-induced DNA synthesis in vascular SMCs may be one possible antiatherogenic mechanism of nifedipine.

References

Berk BC, Brock TA, Webb RC, Taubman MB, Atkinson WJ, Grimbrone MA jr, Alexander RW (1985) Epidermal growth factor, a vascular smooth muscle mitogen, induces rat aortic contraction. J Clin Invest 75:1083–1086

Berridge MJ, Ivine RF (1984) Inositol trisphosphate, a novel second messenger in cellular signal transduction. Nature 312:315–321

Campbell AK (1983) In: Gutfreund H (ed) Intracellular calcium: its universal role as regulator. Wiley, New York

Capponi AM, Lew PP, Vallotton MB (1985) Cytosolic free calcium levels in monolayers of cultured rat aortic smooth muscle cells — effects of angiotensin II and vasopressin. J Biol Chem 260:7386–7842

Etingin OR, Hajjar DP (1985) Nifedipine increases cholesteryl ester hydrolytic activity in lipid-laden rabbit arterial smooth muscle cells. A possible mechanism for its antiatherogenic effect. J Clin Invest 75:1554–1558

Henry PD, Bentley KI (1981) Suppression of atherogenesis in cholesterol-fed rabbit treated with nifedipine. J Clin Invest 68:1366–1369

Hesketh TR, Moore JP, Morris JDH (1985) A common sequence of calcium and pH signals in the mitogenic stimulation of eukaryotic cells. Nature 313:481–484

Kramsch DM, Aspen AJ, Apstein CS (1980) Suppression of experimental atherosclerosis by the Ca^{2+}-antagonist lanthanum. J Clin Invest 65:967–981

Nakao J, Ito H, Oyama T, Chang WC, Murota S (1983) Calcium dependency of aortic smooth muscle cell migration induced by 12-1-hydroxy-5, 8, 10, 14-eicosatetraenoic acid. Atherosclerosis 46:309–319

Rosenblum, IY, Flora L, Eisenstein R (1975) The effect of disodium ethane-1-hydroxy-1, 1-disphosphonate (EHDP) on a rabbit model of atheroarteriosclerosis. Atherosclerosis 22:411–424

Ross R (1971) The smooth muscle cell, Part 2 (growth of smooth muscle in culture and formation of elastic fibers) J Cell Biol 50:172–186

Ross R (1986) The pathogenesis of atherosclerosis; an update. N Engl J Med 314:488–500

Ross R, Glomset JA (1976) The pathogenesis of atherosclerosis. N Engl J Med 295:420–425

Ross R, Glomset JA, Kariya B, Harker LA (1974) A platelet-dependent serum factor that stimulates the proliferation of arterial smooth muscle cells in vitro. Proc Nat Acad Sci USA 71:1207–1210

Stein O, Leitersdorf E, Stein Y (1985) Verapamil enhances receptor-mediated endocytosis of low density lipoproteins by aortic cells in culture. Arteriosclerosis 5:35–44

Tsien RY, Pozzan T, Rink TJ (1982) Calcium homeostasis in intact lymphocytes: cytoplasmic free calcium monitored with a new, intracellularly trapped fluorescent indicator. J Cell Biol 94:325–334

Hypertension

Studies on the Mechanism of the Antihypertensive Effect of Long-Term Administered Nifedipine in Patients with Benign Essential Hypertension

O. Iimura[1], K. Shimamoto[1], and K. Kikuchi[1]

Introduction

The calcium channel blocker nifedipine is a potent relaxant of the arteriolar smooth muscle, producing vasodilatation and thus reducing peripheral resistance and arterial pressure (Guazzi et al. 1977; Robinson et al. 1980). A satisfactory chronic reduction in arterial pressure following the administration of this drug has been demonstrated in hypertensive subjects (Kiowski et al. 1983; Murphy et al. 1983). However, the explanations for the mechanism of the depressor effect of this calcium channel blocker have been based mainly on the results obtained in animal experiments, and detailed mechanism of the depressor action of nifedipine has not yet been clarified, particularly in the clinical field. Moreover, the mechanism of the inhibitory action of nifedipine on aldosterone secretion and the effect of this drug on uric acid metabolism still remains unclear.

To elucidate the mechanisms in which nifedipine clearly reduces blood pressure and exerts an influence on aldosterone secretion and uric acid metabolism in patients with essential hypertension, clinical studies were performed in inpatients with mild to moderate essential hypertension.

Patients and Methods

Patients

All patients with uncomplicated, mild to moderate essential hypertension employed in this study were admitted to our hospital. The patients were either untreated or had discontinued antihypertensive drugs immediately after admission. They were kept on a regular daily diet containing 120 mEq sodium and 75 mEq potassium and were administered a placebo of nifedipine.

[1] Second Department of Internal Medicine, Sapporo Medical College, Sapporo, Japan

The examinations were started after 2 weeks rest following admission, when the blood pressure slightly and spontaneously fell and then stabilized (Iimura et al. 1980).

Methods

Long-Term Administration of Nifedipine: In nine patients with essential hypertension, nifedipine (slow-release tablet Adalat, 60 mg/day, three times per day) was administered for 4 weeks. Daily urine samples were collected 2 days before the start of nifedipine treatment and every day during nifedipine administration. In the early morning after overnight fasting, blood sampling and determination of renal clearance were performed before and 1 week and 4 weeks following the administration of nifedipine.

Effect of Long-Term Administration of Nifedipine on Serum Uric Acid Level in Outpatients: In addition to evaluating the uric acid metabolism in inpatients, the serum uric acid levels were observed before and in average 14 months after nifedipine treatment in 13 outpatients with mild to moderate essential hypertension.

Effect of Nifedipine on Aldosterone Secretion: In seven patients with essential hypertension, nifedipine (60 mg/day, three times per day) was administered for a period of 10 days. Before and 7–10 days after nifedipine administration, 2-h ambulation, angiotensin II infusion, and ACTH injection were performed in these patients. In 2-h ambulation, blood samples were collected before and after the ambulation. In the angiotensin II infusion study, angiotensin II (2.5 ng kg^{-1} min^{-1}) was infused for 1 h. The blood was sampled before and after the infusion. In the ACTH injection study, all patients were pretreated with 0.5 mg dexamethasone 12 h before the examination. Then, 0.25 mg ACTH was injected, and blood samples were collected before and 30, 60 and 90 min after the injection.

Analytical Methods: In this study, mean arterial pressure (MAP); heart rate (HR); plasma noradrenalin (pNA), renin activity (PRA), angiotensin II (pAT-II), aldosterone concentration (PAC), uric acid, creatinine, sodium, and inorganic phosphorus; urine volume (UV), and urinary excretion of sodium (UNaV), uric acid (UUAV), dopamine (uDA), kallikrein (uKAL), kinin (uKIN), and prostaglandin E_2 (PGE_2); fractional excretion of sodium (FENa), inorganic phosphorus (FEP), and uric acid (FEUA); and creatinine clearance (Ccr) were all determined. Moreover, plasma volume (PV), body weight, MAP, and HR responses to infused noradrenalin (0.2 μg kg^{-1} min^{-1}), to infused angiotensin II (10 ng kg^{-1} min^{-1}), and to 60° head-up tilting were also estimated before and 1 week and 4 weeks following the administration of nifedipine.

Blood pressure was measured by the auscultatory method with a standard mercury sphygmomanometer. MAP was calculated as diastolic pressure plus one-third of the pulse pressure. HR was measured from the ECG taken simultaneously. PNA and uDA were determined by high-performance liquid chromatography with an electrochemical detector. PRA (Haber et al. 1969), pAT-II (Shimamoto et al. 1984), PAC, uKAL (Shimamoto et al. 1980), uKIN (Shimamoto et al. 1978), and uPGE$_2$ (Nishimiya et al. 1986) were all measured by the radioimmunoassay method. Blood and urinary sodium, inorganic phosphorus, uric acid, and creatinine were determined by the method of ion electrode, by the method of Kageyama (1971) and by the method of Jaffe (Borsnes and Taussky 1945), respectively. The measurement of FENa, FEP, FEUA, and Ccr were performed according to the clearance method. PV was determined by the ^{125}I-labeled RISA dilution methods (Tarazi et al. 1968), and it was expressed in percent of the mean value per height of normal men and women (ml/cm-% normal). Blood pressure response to noradrenalin and angiotensin II was estimated by the increase in mean arterial pressure responding to intravenous infusion of 0.2 μg kg^{-1} min^{-1} noradrenaline and 10 ng kg^{-1} min^{-1} angiotensin II, respectively.

Statistical Analysis: Statistical analysis was performed by employing analysis of variance and Student's *t* test, where appropriate, for paired or unpaired data. Correlation was calculated using linear regression analysis. Each of the values were presented as mean ± 1 SEM.

Results

Long-Term Administration of Nifedipine

The effects of long-term administration of nifedipine on hemodynamics, renal functions, and endocrinological parameters are shown in Table 1.

Following the administration of nifedipine, MAP was reduced significantly from 121±3 mmHg to 105±4 mmHg at 1 week and to 94±3 mmHg at 4 weeks, while HR did not change significantly. PNA increased slightly but significantly at 1 week, while not at 4 weeks. Both PRA and pAT-II were clearly elevated at 1 week and 4 weeks. However, despite the remarkable elevation of pAT-II, PAC represented no significant increase following nifedipine administration. No significant changes in uDA, uKAL, uKIN, or uPGE$_2$ were observed following this drug.

The effects of nifedipine on renal function are shown in Table 1 and Fig. 1. Values for UV, UNaV, FENa, and FEP did not present any change at the points of 1 week and 4 weeks after nifedipine administration (Table 1). However, UV, UNaV (Fig. 1), and FENa were markedly augmented by nifedipine for 2–3 days immediately after treatment and nearly returned to the control value at 1 week after the beginning of drug administration (Fig. 1). Thus, a significant decrease was observed in PV at 1 week and in body weight at 1 week and 4 weeks following nifedipine. No change was found in Ccr throughout this course following nifedipine administration.

Table 1. Effect of long-term administered nifedipine on hemodynamics, water sodium metabolism and pressor and depressor systems

	n	Before	1 week	4 weeks
Mean arterial pressure (mm Hg)	9	121±3	105±4[d]	97±3[d]
Heart rate (beats/min)	9	63±2	66±2	64±2
Plasma volume (ml/cm-% normal)	9	99.5±7.9	91.3±7.0[b]	92.2±8.7
Body weight (kg)	9	63.9±3.1	63.3±3.1[c]	62.5±2.8[b]
Urine volume (ml/min)	9	3.92±0.51	4.05±0.33	3.84±0.37
Urinary sodium excretion (μEq/min)	9	114±14	158±26[a]	133±32
Fractional excretion of sodium (%)	9	1.02±0.18	1.35±0.28[a]	1.30±0.32
Fractional excretion of inorganic phosphorus (%)	9	15.2±2.3	15.8±2.0	14.2±1.8
Creatinine clearance (ml/min)	9	77.3±533	86.2±8.6	80.2±6.7
Plasma noradrenalin (pg/ml)	9	161.0±13.8	215.0±26.9[b]	161.2±24.1
Plasma renin activity (ng/ml per hour)	9	0.61±0.17	1.16±0.36[b]	1.20±0.24[d]
Plasma angiotensin II (pg/ml)	7	6.2±4.4	9.5±5.9[b]	11.9±8.1[b]
Plasma aldosterone concentration (pg/ml)	8	120.1±30.8	110.0±26.2	108.0±35.4
Urinary dopamine (ng/min)	9	192.0±13.1	162.1±10.5	155.3±19.7
Urinary kallikrein (ng/min)	8	97.6±18.1	108.0±21.8	96.0±18.0
Urinary kinin (ng/min)	9	9.3±1.6	12.5±3.2[a]	9.5±1.6
Urinary prostaglandin E_2 (pg/min)	7	74.7±14.0	59.6±18.5	75.7±22.6

Mean ± SEM
[a] $p<0.1$
[b] $p<0.05$
[c] $p<0.01$
[d] $p<0.001$

In the study of 60° head-up tilting, MAP before the tilting decreased significantly at 1 week and 4 weeks following nifedipine, and MAP after the tilting also tended to be lowered as compared to those observed before the administration of nifedipine. By the tilting manuever, MAP elevated significantly before and at 1 week following this drug treatment, but not significantly at 4 weeks. The elevation of MAP by the tilting manuever was significantly lower at 4 weeks following nifedipine (−0.4±3.4 mmHg) than that before drug administration (7.9±2.3 mmHg). HR was significantly increased by the tilting manuever before and following nifedipine, but no significant difference was observed in these increases before or at 1 week or 4 weeks following this drug. Basal pNA revealed a significant increase at 1 week, and the tilting manuever resulted in a significant increase of pNA before and at 1 week and 4 weeks following nifedipine. However, these increases of pNA by the tilting showed no significant difference before or 1 week or 4 weeks following this drug.

The effect of nifedipine administration on responses of MAP and HR to infused noradrenalin or to angiotensin II is demonstrated in Fig. 2. Both the response of MAP and that of HR to infused noradrenalin were significantly lower at 1 week and 4 weeks following nifedipine administration than before this drug. On the other hand, the ratio of ΔHR/ΔMAP showed a lower tendency at 4 weeks than that before nifedipine. The response of MAP to in-

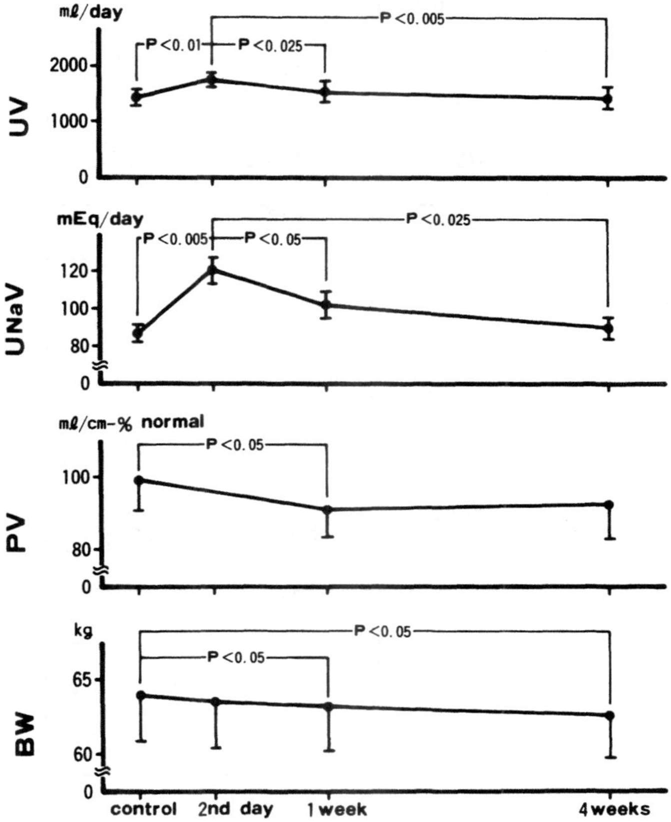

Fig. 1. Long-term effects of nifedipine on urine volume *(UV)*, urinary sodium excretion *(UNaV)*, plasma volume *(PV)*, and body weight *(BW)* in essential hypertensives

fused angiotensin II was significantly lower at 1 week and 4 weeks following nifedipine than that before this drug, while no significant difference was observed between ΔHR responding to angiotensin II before nifedipine and that at 1 week or 4 weeks following this drug. The ratio ΔHR/ΔMAP responded to angiotensin II tended to be suppressed at 4 weeks following nifedipine compared to that in the control period.

Figure 3 presents the effect of nifedipine on serum uric acid levels in nine inpatients and 13 outpatients with essential hypertension. Serum uric acid levels were decreased significantly at 1 week and 4 weeks following nifedipine as compared to the control levels in inpatients. In outpatients, serum uric acid levels were decreased significantly at 14 months following nifedipine. The effect of nifedipine on Ccr, UUAV, and FENa in these inpatients is demonstrated in Fig. 4. While no significant change was found in Ccr during these periods, FEUA increased significantly at 1 week following nifedipine, and the same tendency was observed at 4 weeks. Moreover, significantly positive cor-

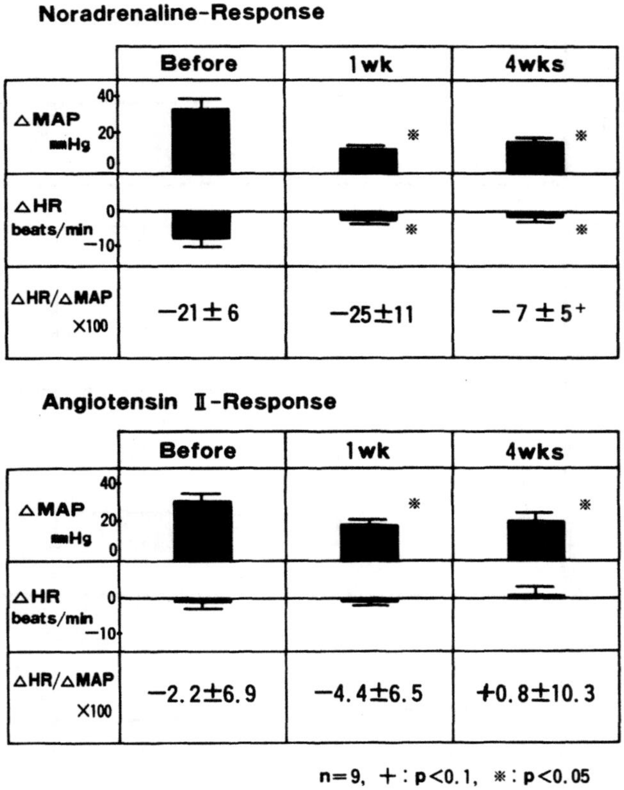

Fig. 2. Effects of long-term administered nifedipine on responses of mean arterial pressure *(ΔMAP)* and heart rate *(ΔHR)* to infused noradrenalin (0.2 μg kg^{-1} min^{-1}) or to angiotensin II (10 ng kg^{-1} min^{-1}) in essential hypertensives

relations were recognized between the change of FEUA (ΔFEUA) and that of FENa (ΔFENa) or FEP (ΔFEP) when both data at 1 week and 4 weeks were used (Fig. 5).

Effect of Nifedipine on Aldosterone Secretion

The effect of nifedipine on PRA and PAC responding to the ambulation for 2 h in essential hypertensives are shown in Fig. 6. After ambulation, both PRA and PAC clearly increased before treatment and at 10 days following nifedipine administration. This increase of PRA was significantly higher following nifedipine administration than that before this drug, while no difference was found in the change of PAC which responded to ambulation before and after nifedipine. Figure 7 presents the effect of nifedipine on PAC response to infused angiotensin II (2.5 ng kg^{-1} min^{-1} for 1 h) in essential hypertensives.

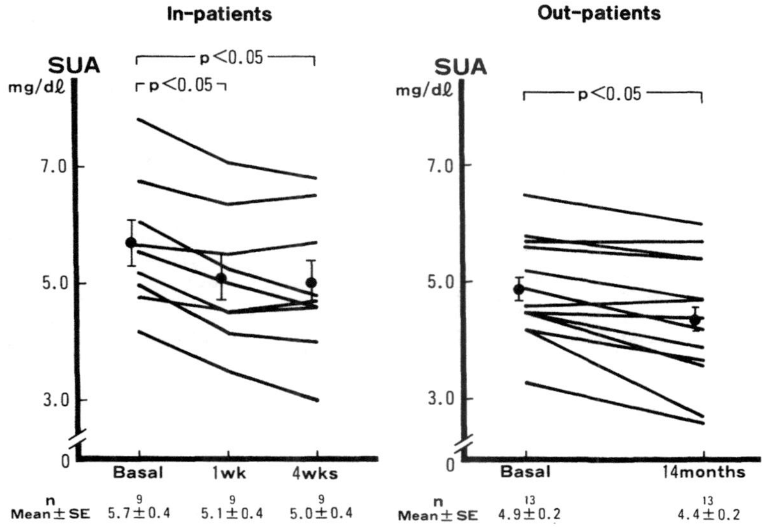

Fig. 3. Effect of nifedipine on serum uric acid *(SUA)* in essential hypertensives

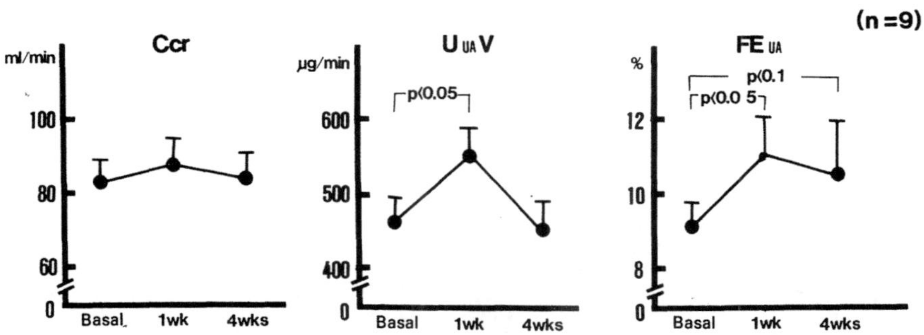

Fig. 4. Effects of nifedipine on creatinine clearance *(Ccr),* urinary excretion of uric acid *(UUAV),* and fractional excretion of uric acid *(FEUA)* in essential hypertensives

PAC increased significantly before and after nifedipine, but this increase in PAC was significantly lower following nifedipine compared to that before drug administration. The effect of nifedipine on the PAC response to injected ACTH (0.25 mg, i.v.) in these patients is demonstrated in Fig. 8. Both before and after nifedipine administration, PAC increased significantly at 30, 60, and 90 min after the injection of ACTH. However, no significant difference could be detected when comparing the change of PAC responding to ACTH before nifedipine and that following this drug.

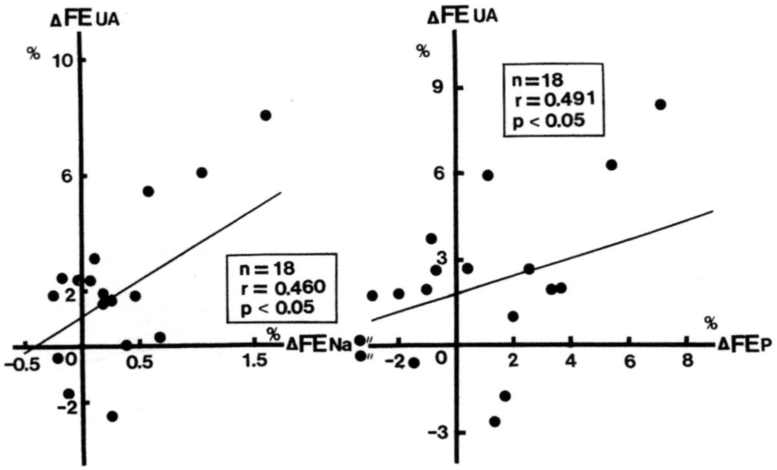

Fig. 5. Correlations between ΔFENa and ΔFEUA or between ΔFEP and ΔFEUA following nifedipine administration in essential hypertensives

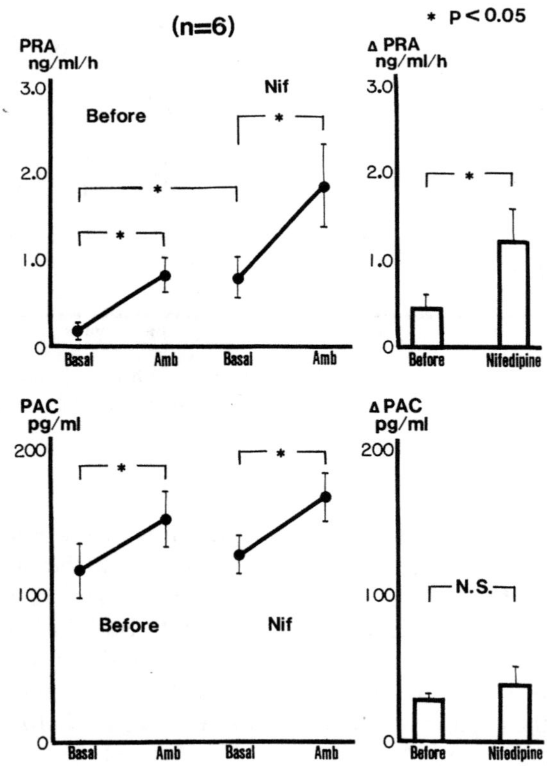

Fig. 6. Effects of nifedipine (*Nif*) on renin and aldosterone responses to ambulation for 2 h in essential hypertensives

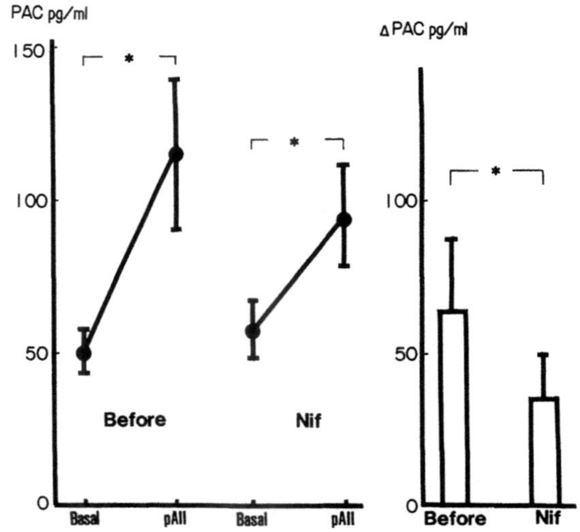

Fig. 7. Effect of nifedipine *(Nif)* on aldosterone response to angiotensin II infusion (2.5 ng kg^{-1} min^{-1} for 1 h in essential hypertensives ($n=7$); * $p<0.05$

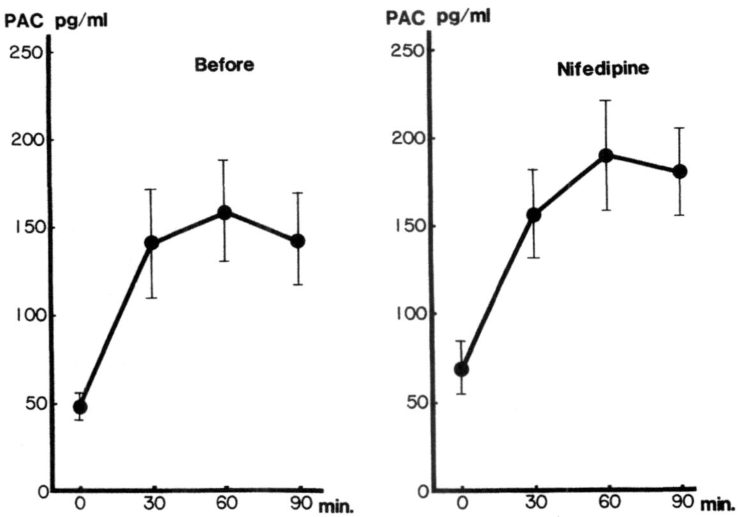

Fig. 8. Effect of nifedipine on aldosterone response to injected ACTH (0.25 mg i.v.) in essential hypertensives ($n=7$)

Discussion

In recent years, nifedipine, a calcium channel blocker, has been used successfully to lower blood pressure in hypertension. This effect seems to be due mainly to vasodilation caused by interference with the excitation-contraction coupling in peripheral resistance vessels (Grun and Fleckenstein 1972).

In this study, to elucidate the mechanism by which nifedipine clearly reduces blood pressure in essential hypertensives, the effects of long-term nifedipine treatment on hemodynamics, renal function, sympathetic nerve activity, the renin-angiotensin-aldosterone system, and uric acid metabolism were investigated in inpatients with mild to moderate essential hypertension.

From this study, it was shown that body weight and PV decreased significantly following nifedipine administration. The mechanisms behind these findings are apparent from this study, in which reductions in body weight and PV were shown to be caused by the augmentation of diuresis and natriuresis in the relatively acute phase of nifedipine treatment. Maintenance of the control level of diuresis and natriuresis in the chronic phase of this drug treatment took place as a result of nifedipine administration. The antihypertensive effects of peripheral vasodilators are often limited by counterregulatory mechanisms, including sodium and water retention. However, as described above, nifedipine does not have such counterregulatory mechanism. Therefore, the diuretic and natriuretic actions of nifedipine may augment the hypotensive effect of this drug in long-term treatment. The detailed mechanism of diuresis and natriuresis by nifedipine remains unclear, although the increase in renal blood flow may contribute to some extent.

Following nifedipine administration, pNA increased significantly at 1 week with a marked fall in blood pressure but not at 4 weeks despite the same fall in blood pressure. Moreover, HR did not change following the administration of this drug in long-term treatment. These data suggest that nifedipine partly inhibits sympathetic nerve activity and may blunt the arterial baroreflexes in essential hypertensives in long-term treatment. In fact, the sympathetic nerve activity induced by the tilting manuever was markedly suppressed following nifedipine administration, as shown in the decreased MAP response and pNA response to tilting manuever following nifedipine at 4 weeks. In addition, the suppressed arterial baroreflexes by nifedipine might be confirmed by the response to infused noradrenalin and to angiotensin II in essential hypertensives, suggested by the decreasing tendency of $\Delta HR/\Delta MAP$ following nifedipine compared to that of pretreatment state. From these results, it should be considered that both interference with sympathetic function and blunted arterial baroreflexes may contribute, at least in part, to the depressor mechanism of nifedipine.

Next, the effect of nifedipine on aldosterone secretion should be discussed. It has been reported that nifedipine elevates PRA in essential hypertensives (Aoki et al. 1978; Olivari et al. 1979; Pedersen et al. 1979). On the other hand, it is widely recognized that angiotensin II stimulates aldosterone secretion from adrenal glands, and that the increase of factors having direct or indirect effect on PRA, in general, might be thought to result in a comparable increase of PAC. If this is the case, one may expect an increase not only in PRA and pAT-II but also in PAC in patients treated with nifedipine. However, this speculated sequence of events has not been observed in our study, as shown by no change of basal PAC in spite of a marked increase of basal PRA and pAT-II after the long-term nifedipine administration. Angiotensin II, potassium, and ACTH are the known primary stimulators of aldosterone secretion from the zona glomerulosa. Regarding the mechanism in which nifedipine might inhibit aldosterone secretion, in the studies of the 2-h ambulation, angiotensin II infusion, and ACTH injection, evidence was obtained that nifedipine attenuates the aldosterone secretion responding to angiotensin II, but not ACTH. However, it was not clarified in this study whether nifedipine inhibits the potassium-induced aldosterone release or not. It is possible that the hypotensive effect of nifedipine in long-term use is due in part to the inhibition of aldosterone secretion from adrenal glands.

On the other hand, the effects of antihypertensive drugs on lipids, glucose, and uric acid metabolism have recently created interest due to the inevitable long-term treatment of these drugs, and caution has been raised in the case of some antihypertensive drugs, including diuretics and β-blockers. However, the effect of nifedipine on uric acid metabolism has not been clarified yet. In this study, it was found that nifedipine significantly decreases the serum uric acid levels in both inpatients for 4 weeks and outpatients for 13 months of treatment. The mechanism of the decrease of serum uric acid may be explained by the increase in UUAV, because both UUAV and FEUA were augmented significantly following nifedipine. Moreover, the change in FEUA correlated significantly with the change in FENa and that in FEP, suggesting that the increase in UUAV may be caused by the inhibition of uric acid reabsorption in proximal tubules of nephrone as well as sodium. It is still unclear whether nifedipine has some direct effect on uric acid metabolism, although the increased renal blood flow may be partly connected to this augmented excretion of uric acid in urine by a similar mechanism as that of sodium.

In conclusion, it was suggested that the hypotensive mechanism of nifedipine may be related to the interference with sympathetic function, suppression or resetting of arterial baroreflexes function, augmentation of diuresis and natriuresis, and suppression of aldosterone secretion responding to angiotensin II, in addition to the direct dilatation of the arterial beds. It was also demonstrated in this study that nifedipine might improve the uric acid metabolism in patients with mild to moderate essential hypertension.

References

Aoki K, Kondo S, Mochizuki A, Yoshida T, Kato S, Kato K, Takikawa K (1978) Antihypertensive effect of cardiovascular Ca^{++}-antagonist in hypertensive patients in the absence and presence of beta-adrenergic blockade. Jpn Heart J 96:218–226

Borsnes RW, Taussky HH (1945) On the colorimetric determination of creatinine by the Jaffe reaction. Biol Chem 158:581–591

Grun G, Fleckenstein A (1972) Die elektromechanische Entkoppelung der glatten Gefäßmuskulatur als Grundprinzip der Coronardilatation durch 4-(2′-nitrophenyl)-2,6-dimethyl-1,4-dihydropyridin-3,5-dicarbonsaare -dimethylester (Bay a 1040, nifedipine). Arzneimittelforschung 22:334–344

Guazzi M, Oliveri MT, Polese A, Fiorentini C, Magrini F, Moruzzi P (1977) Nifedipine, a new antihypertensive with rapid action. Clin Pharmacol Ther 22:528–532

Haber E, Koerner Y, Page LB, Kliman B, Purnode A (1969) Application of a radioimmunoassay for angiotensin I to the physiological measurements of plasma renin activity in normal human subjects. J Clin Endocrinol 29:1349–1355
Iimura O, Kikuchi K, Miyama A, Nakao T, Kondo A, Takigami Y, Miyahara M (1980) Studies on sympathetic nerve, renin-angiotensin and renal kallikrein-kinin systems and water-sodium balance in essential hypertension. Jpn Circ J 44:411–421
Kageyama N (1971) A direct colorimetric determination of uric acid in serum and urine with uricase-catalase system. Clin Chim Acta 31:421–426
Kiowski W, Bertel O, Erne P, Bolli P, Hulthen UL, Rith R, Buhler FR (1983) Hemodynamic and reflex responses to acute and chronic antihypertensive therapy with the calcium entry blocker nifedipine. Hypertension 5 [Suppl I]:I-70-74
Murphy MB, Scriven AJL, Dollery CT (1983) Role of nifedipine in treatment of hypertension. Br Med J 287:257–259
Nishimiya T, Shimamoto K, Tanaka S, Ura N, Mita T, Nakagawa M, Maeda T, Yamaguchi Y, Masuda A, Iimura O (1986) The role of renal kallikrein-kinin system and prostaglandins in diuresis and natriuresis following saline infusion in normotensives and essential hypertensives. Adv Exp Med Biol 198 B:337–342
Olivari MT, Bartorelli C, Polese A, Fiorentini C, Moruzzi P, Guazzi MD (1979) Treatment of hypertension with nifedipine, a calcium antagonist agent. Circulation 59:1056–1062
Pedersen OL, Mikkelsen E, Christensin NJ, Kornerup HJ, Pedersen EB (1979) Effects of nifedipine on plasma renin, aldosterone and catecholamines in arterial hypertension. Eur J Clin Pharmacol 21:235–240
Robinson BF, Dodds, RJ, Kelsey CR (1980) Effects of nifedipine on resistance vessels, arteries and veins in man. Br J Clin Pharmacol 10:433–438
Shimamoto K, Ando T, Nakao T, Tanaka S, Sakuma M, Miyahara M (1978) A sensitive radioimmunoassay method for urinary kinins in man. J Lab Clin Med 91:721–728
Shimamoto K, Chao J, Margolius HS (1980) The radioimmunoassay of human urinary kallikrein and comparison with kallikrein activity measurements. J Clin Endocrinol Metab 51:840–848
Shimamoto K, Ishida H, Nakahashi Y, Nishitani T, Hosoda S, Yokoyama T, Tanaka S, Iimura O (1984) A very sensitive direct radioimmunoassay system for plasma angiotensin II and its clinical application in various hypertensive diseases. Jpn Circ J 48:1228–1235
Tarazi RC, Frohlich ED, Dustan HP (1968) Plasma volume in men with essential hypertension. N Engl J Med 278:762–765

Nifedipine Retard as Monotherapy for Essential Hypertension: A Randomized Controlled Cross-over Study

K. S. Woo[1], C. O. Pun[1], and J. Vallance-Owen[1]

Introduction

Over the past couple of decades diuretics, methyldopa, and β-blockers have been the common drugs used as first-line regimen for treating hypertension [1–3]. Some large-scale long-term studies, however, have unmasked certain side effects of the diuretics and β-blockers, and they were seen not to be well tolerated in certain patients [4–9]. These findings have stimulated interest in the search for alternative regimens. Calcium antagonists have been found to be safe and effective in treating hypertensive crisis as well as resistant hypertension, although experience is still limited regarding its application as a first-step monotherapy regimen in hypertension [10–11]. With the availability of a long-acting preparation of nifedipine that is more convenient for users, the application of nifedipine as a first-line drug for treating mild to moderate hypertension may prove desirable and appealing [12–13].

This chapter reports on our experience using nifedipine retard as monotherapy in essential hypertension as compared to a β-blocker

Patients and Methods

Forty patients with mild to moderate essential hypertension seen in the hypertension clinic of the Prince of Wales Hospital (Hong Kong) in the period from September 1985 to December 1986 were recruited. There were 19 men and 21 women; ages ranged from 32 to 70 years (mean 55.6 ± 10.8). Inclusion criteria were:

(a) mild to moderate hypertension with blood pressure (BP) of 160/95–220/120 mmHg for at least three readings;
(b) age younger than 70 years;
(c) absence of systemic complication, including cardiac, renal, or cerebrovascular involvement; and
(d) essential hypertension.

[1] Department of Medicine, The Chinese University of Hong Kong, Prince of Wales Hospital, Shatin, NT, Hong Kong

Those with underlying etiological causes, severe hypertension (BP<220/120 mmHg), or contraindication for β-blockers were excluded.

During each visit, BP was measured by a random zero sphygmomanometer in sitting position after 5 min rest and in standing position after 2 min. Korotkoff phase 5 was taken as the diastolic BP, and the average of three readings was recorded for each posture.

After a washout period of 4 weeks, patients were randomized into group A taking metoprolol (50–100 mg b.i.d.) or group B taking nifedipine retard (20–40 mg b.i.d.) for 4 weeks with the object of normalizing BP in the range 130/70–160/90 mmHg. This was followed by another washout period of 2 weeks after which subjects were crossed over to the other drug. Patients were given a nifedipine retard placebo tablet twice per day during both washout periods. A treadmill exercise was performed at the end of the study while they were maintained on either of the two drugs.

ECG, chest X ray, and biochemical profile were repeated during each treatment period. During each visit, any adverse symptom was recorded in detail.

Four patients with normalization of BP during placebo period were excluded. Two patients requiring withdrawal due to adverse symptoms were excluded from the analysis of BP response, but they were included for the analysis of adverse side effects.

The χ-test with Yates' corredtion was used to assess the statistical significance of adverse reactions [14].

Results

BP levels are shown in Table 1. Good BP control was achieved in 89.4% patients on nifedipine with a mean daily dose of 51.2 mg compared to 60.5% of

Table 1. Blood pressure (mm Hg) in different periods

	First phase		Second phase	
	Placebo (weeks 1–4)	Drug (weeks 5–8)	Placebo (weeks 9, 10)	Drug (weeks 11–14)
Group A (M/N)				
Before	175.8 ± 22.8	167.3 ± 28.0	177.4 ± 32.7	153.5 ± 22.3[a]
After	101.0 ± 5.7	92.9 ± 9.7	100.6 ± 12.0	89.2 ± 8.1[b]
Group B (N/M)				
Before	178.3 ± 18.0	144.1 ± 15.7	170.9 ± 23.7	158.9 ± 20.5[a]
After	101.6 ± 8.1	87.2 ± 10.0	98.5 ± 10.3	87.5 ± 11.6[b]
*p**	>0.5	<0.05	>0.1	<0.05[a] >0.1[b]

M, Metoprolol; N, nifedipine.
* Group A versus group B.

patients on metoprolol with mean daily dose of 160 mg (Table 2). The mean BP during nifedipine was significantly lower than that during metoprolol (Table 3). During treadmill exercise, maximal BP in the two groups was similar (Table 4). No significant postural variations were seen in BP, but standing pulse rates were slightly higher in the nifedipine and placebo periods (Table 5). Adverse symptoms were reported in 33% of patients on nifedipine com-

Table 2. Blood pressure control

	Metoprolol	Nifedipine
Excellent (≤150/90)	11 (28.9%)	20 (52.6%)
Good (150/90–160/95)	12 (31.6%)	14 (36.8%)
Overall	23 (60.5%)	34 (89.4%)
Mean systolic (mm Hg)	165.5 ± 27.0	148.8 ± 21.9
Difference (95% CI)	16.7 (4.7–28.7)[a]	
Mean diastolic (mm Hg)	92.7 ± 10.2	87.8 ± 11.6
Difference (95% CI)	5.4 (1.4–9.4)[b]	

CI, Cardiac index.
[a] $p<0.001$
[b] $p<0.01$

Table 3. Blood pressure response during treadmill exercise

	Metoprolol	Nifedipine	p
At rest	158.4/86.9	161.8/88.2	>0.1
Exercise	189.3/93.7	191.8/94.2	>0.1

Table 4. Mean blood pressure (mm Hg) in different postures

	Placebo		Metoprolol	Nifedipine
	First	Second		
Systolic				
Lying	175.8 ± 17.4	175.2 ± 25.3	166.2 ± 25.7	151.5 ± 16.5
Sitting	176.1 ± 17.2	171.9 ± 29.0	163.8 ± 23.6	149.4 ± 16.6
Standing	178.3 ± 16.5	170.4 ± 16.3	165.0 ± 10.2	150.8 ± 10.1
p	>0.1	>0.05	>0.1	>0.1
Diastolic				
Lying	100.1 ± 6.9	100.4 ± 10.1	93.2 ± 9.9	89.1 ± 8.1
Sitting	101.7 ± 7.2	99.1 ± 10.4	93.1 ± 9.4	87.9 ± 10.0
Standing	101.7 ± 6.2	100.1 ± 8.6	91.7 ± 4.7	87.5 ± 7.5
p	>0.05	>0.5	>0.1	>0.5

Table 5. Pulse rate

	Placebo**		Metoprolol	Nifedipine**
	First	Second		
Lying	76.5±6.7	74.6± 9.3	67.1±8.2	77.9±10.9
Sitting	76.7±7.3	75.1±10.1	66.8±7.6	77.6±11.2
Standing	85.1±5.2	80.0± 3.1	63.3±8.1	82.0±12.1
p	>0.5*	>0.5	>0.5	>0.5
	<0.001+	<0.05	>0.1	>0.1

** $p>0.1$
* Lying versus sitting.
+ Lying versus standing.
** Placebo versus nifedipine.

Table 6. Side effects

	Placebo 1 ($n=45$)	Placebo 2 ($n=43$)	Metoprolol ($n=42$)	Nifedipine ($n=42$)
Gastrointestinal	3 (7%)	0 (0%)	4 (10%)	3 (7%)
Flushing	1 (2%)	0 (0%)	0 (0%)	2 (5%)
Edema	0 (0%)	0 (0%)	0 (0%)	4 (10%)
Headache	10 (22%)	*7 (16%)	2 (5%)	10 (24%)
Dizziness	8 (18%)	3 (7%)	3 (7%)	6 (14%)
Tiredness	3 (7%)	1 (2%)	4 (10%)	2 (5%)
Palpitation	2 (4%)	1 (2%)	1 (2%)	*3 (7%)
Others	11 (24%)	5 (12%)	8 (19%)	12 (28%)
Withdrawal	0	*1 (2%)	0	*1 (2%)
Nil none	30 (67%)	30 (70%)	36 (86%)	28 (67%)

Table 7. Biochemical and radiological profiles

	Placebo		Metoprolol	Nifedipine
	First	Second		
Potassium	3.9±0.4	4.0±0.5	4.1±0.5	3.7±0.3
Calcium	2.4±0.1	2.4±0.9	2.3±0.1	2.4±0.1
Urea	5.9±1.4	6.3±1.5	6.3±1.5	6.3±1.5
Creatinine*	81.0±21.7	81.7±13.5	81.7±16.7	78.6±20.4
Urate	0.37±0.09	0.39±0.08	0.39±0.08	0.37±0.07
Glucose	5.2±1.3	5.2±1.0	5.1±1.1	5.1±1.0
Cholesterol	5.9±1.0	5.5±1.3	5.1±1.3	5.5±1.1
Chest X-ray**	51.0±3.9	51.8±1.6	52.5±3.7	49.2±3.4

p (Nifedipine versus placebo) > 0.1.
* μmol/L; ** % of cardiothoracic ratio; all others: in mmol/L.

pared to 14% on metoprolol ($p<0.05$) and 30%–33% on placebo ($p<0.5$; Table 6), including face flushing, ankle edema, dizziness, and palpitation, most of which were well tolerated. Headache was a common complaint and was present in 16%–24% of patients during the placebo and nifedipine periods. Withdrawal of drugs was required on two occasions, in a woman taking nifedipine due to palpitation and in a man on placebo due to headache. There were no significant differences in renal function or other biochemical profiles in the two groups (Table 7).

Discussion

The present study confirms nifedipine retard to be an effective and more potent antihypertensive drug as compared with the commonly used β-blocker metoprolol. Used as monotherapy, it was effective in 89.4% of patients with mild to moderate essential hypertension. Addition of a diuretic or a β-blocker is often effective in normalizing BP in the remaining 10% of patients. Adverse symptoms were often transient, and the majority of these were reasonably well tolerated. The twice daily regimen of this long-acting nifedipine preparation is more convenient than the plain capsule, and patient compliance is therefore greater. However, it is more expensive than other common first-step medications, and this could affect its wider applications as first-step monotherapy in many Asian-Pacifix countries where resources are still limited. A greater therapeutic prospect of calcium antagonist as first-step regimen may be present where there are coexisting diseases, such as ischemic heart disease, chronic obstructive airway disease, left ventricular failure, or peripheral vascular disease, where its beneficial action on the cardiac or smooth muscles is particularly appealing.

Acknowledgement: The authors wish to thank Bayer China Co. Ltd. (Hong Kong) for the supply of nifedipine and placebo tablets and provision of computer service.

References

1. National Institute of Health (1973) Executive summary of the task force reports to the Hypertension Information and Education Advisory Committee. In: National high blood pressure education program, Bethesda, National Institute of Health, Washington, pp1–20
2. Grimm RH, Luephker RV, Taylor H, Blackburn H (1982) Long term effects of a blood pressure survey on patient treatment in a community. Circulation 65:946–950
3. Veterans Administration Cooperative Study Group on Antihypertensive Agents (1982) Comparison of propranolol and hydrochlorothiazide for the initial treatment of hypertension. I. Results of short term titration with emphasis on racial differences in response. JAMA 248:1966–2003
4. Multiple Risk Factor Intervention Trial Research Group (1982) Multiple risk factor intervention trial: risk factor changes and mortality results. JAMA 248:1465–1477

5. Medical Research Council Working Party (1981) Adverse reactions to bendrofluazide and propranolol for the treatment of mild hypertension. Lancet ii:539–544
6. McCarron DA (1984) Diuretic therapy for mild hypertension: the real cost of treatment. Am J Cardiol 53:9A–11A
7. Kaplan NM (1984) Therapy of mild hypertension: an overview. Am J Cardiol 53:2A–8A
8. Opie LH (1984) Drugs and the heart four years on. Lancet i:496–500
9. Koncaid-Smith P (1984) Beta-adrenergic receptor blocking drugs in hypertension. Special reference to their use as initial therapy. Am J Cardiol 53:12A–15A
10. Bayly S, Dobbs RJ, Robinson BF (1982) Nifedipine in the treatment of hypertension: Report of a double-blind controlled trial. Clin Pharmacol 14:509–512
11. Frishman W, Charlap S, Kimmel B et al. (1986) Twice-daily administration of oral Verapamil in the treatment of essential hypertension. Arch Intern Med 46:561-565
12. Hornung Rs, Gould Ba, Jones RI, Sonecha TN, Raftery EB (1983) Nifedipine tablets for systemic hypertension: A study using continuous ambulatory intraarterial recording. Am J Cardiol 51:1323–1327
13. Banzet O, Colin JN, Thibonnier M, Singlas E, Alexandre JM, Corvol P (1983) Acute antihypertensive effect and pharmacokinetics of a tablet preparation of nifedipine. Europ J Clin Pharmacol 24:145–150
14. Swinscow TVD (1976) The chi-square tests. Br Med J 2:291–292

Long-Term Treatment of Hypertensive Patients with Nifedipine Tablet

M. Hiwatari[1], K. Abe[1], K. Yoshinaga[1], T. Saito[2], and S. Sasou[2]

Introduction

Because of its potent vasodilatory effect [1], nifedipine has been well known to lower blood pressure not only in experimental hypertensive animals [2] but also in human hypertensive subjects [3]. However, duration of the hypotensive effect of nifedipine in capsule form is rather short compared with that of other antihypertensive drugs [2]. This requires the daily administration of three or four nifedipine capsules to hypertensive patients to obtain good control of blood pressure levels. To overcome the short duration of action of nifedipine capsule, a retard form of nifedipine, nifedipine tablet, has recently been developed which enables the control of blood pressure through two daily administrations. In the present study, we have examined the efficacy of nifedipine tablet in the long-term treatment of hypertensive patients.

Subjects and Methods

Subjects: The study included 11 patients (five women and six men; mean age, 51.2 years) who had been diagnosed as having essential or renal hypertension in our hypertensive clinic. Four patients had no antihypertensive treatment prior to the study, with systolic/diastolic blood pressure levels of over 160/90 mmHg for at least a 2-week control period. The remaining seven patients had already been treated for their hypertension, but the control of their blood pressure was not satisfactory. The latter group included one patient who had been treated with nifedipine capsule, which was changed to nifedipine tablet because of wide fluctuations in blood pressure. Severe brain ischemia, congestive heart failure, and pregnancy were ruled out before the start of study.

Blood Pressure Measurement and Laboratory Examinations: Prior to the study, blood pressure for at least a 2-week control period was confirmed to be stable; values at the final point of this control period were then adopted as

[1] Second Department of Internal Medicine, Tohoku University School of Medicine, Sendai, Japan
[2] Miyagi National Hospital, Miyagi, Japan

control values for the respective patients. During the study, medicines administered previously were not fundamentally changed. If the doses of antihypertensive drugs could be reduced, firstly we tried to reduce doses of antihypertensive drugs other than nifedipine tablet, finally ceasing administration of nifedipine tablet only if necessary. Nifedipine tablet (20 mg) was given twice daily with an initial dose of 40 mg/day, which was changed according to the level of blood pressure. Measurement of blood pressure was carried out every 2 weeks up to 8 weeks and every month afterward. Before, 8 weeks and 6 months after treatment with nifedipine tablet, laboratory examinations were performed.

Effectiveness: Antihypertensive efficacy of nifedipine tablet was judged from changes in blood pressure from the control values at respective points. Subjective complaints were asked by doctors at each measurement of blood pressure.

Results

Table 1 presents the profiles of the 11 patients in this study. The pathogenesis of hypertension in these patients showed nine cases of essential and two of renal forms. The study period ranged from 9 to 23 months with an average of 13.9 months. Values for blood pressure shown in Table 1 are those just before and 6 months after treatment with nifedipine tablet.

In our preliminary study, we confirmed that oral administration of nifedipine tablet (20 mg) twice daily can ensure sufficient levels of plasma concentration of nifedipine to be able to lower blood pressure. Figure 1 summarizes

Table 1. Patient profiles

Case no.	Sex	Age	Study period (months)	Dose (mg)	Blood pressure		Renal or essential[a]
					Before	After	
1	M	40	9	40	180/96	152/80	E +
2	M	49	18	40/20/40	184/98	140/90	R +
3	F	55	18	40	300/160	180/100	E −
4	M	52	23	40	134/94	130/94	E +
5	F	45	9	40	142/100	120/94	E +
6	M	72	9	40	160/110	120/88	E +
7	M	66	12	40	140/90	120/72	E +
8	F	45	11	40/20	194/110	110/68	E −
9	M	48	13	40/60/40	160/110	98/76	E −
10	F	54	12	40	156/105	120/70	E −
11	F	37	19	40	160/110	120/70	R +

[a] With (+) and without (−) other antihypertensive treatment previously.

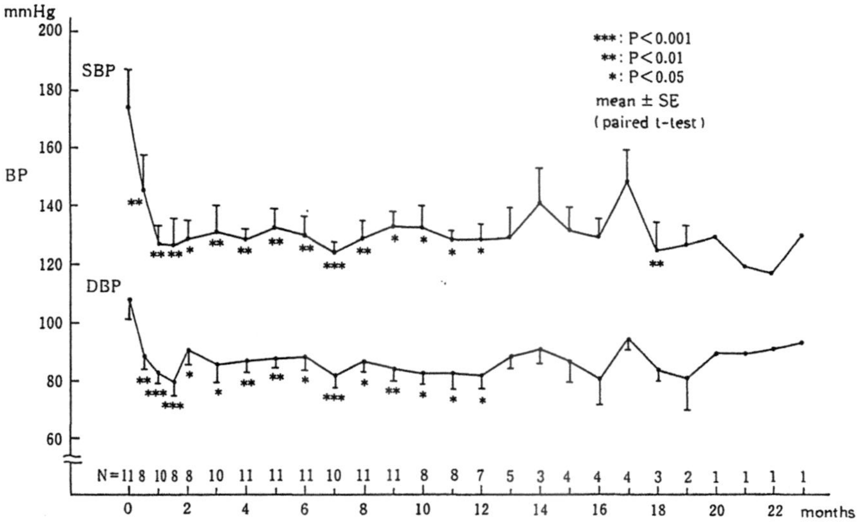

Fig. 1. Changes in systolic *(SBP)* and diastolic blood pressure *(DBP)* during treatment with nifedipine tablet in essential and renal hypertensive patients

changes in systolic and diastolic blood pressure following treatment with nifedipine tablet. Mean values of systolic/diastolic blood pressure fell from 174/108 mmHg to 145/88 mmHg at 2 weeks and to 127/82 mmHg at 4 weeks after treatment, and blood pressure was controlled well thereafter. After 12 months, mean values were below 140/90 mmHg; after 12 months, we could not detect a further significant fall in blood pressure because the number of patients gradually decreased.

Changes in mean arterial pressure are shown in Fig. 2. Mean blood pressure fell markedly at 2 weeks and remained well controlled thereafter in most cases. The horizontal lines in Fig. 2 were drawn at the levels of 117 and 107 mmHg, which were the mean blood pressure levels for 160/95 and 140/90 mmHg, for convenience in assessing the efficacy of hypotensive effects of nifedipine tablet. Most patients showed values for mean blood pressure of below 117 mmHg, and three-fourths of them were below 107 mmHg throughout the study.

Effectiveness of nifedipine tablet in long-term treatment of hypertensive patients was judged from the changes in blood pressure using the criteria shown in Table 2. Nine patients out of the 11 showed apparent falls in blood pressure with these criteria, and three of them could cease or reduce the doses of other antihypertensive drugs. One case in the group without change in blood pressure was a patient being treated with nifedipine capsule (30 mg/day), propranolol (30 mg/day) and clonidine (150 µg/day) previously. After the substitution of nifedipine capsule by nifedipine tablet, doses of propranolol and clonidine were reduced to 20 mg/day and 75 µg/day, respectively, in spite of the lack of change in blood pressure levels.

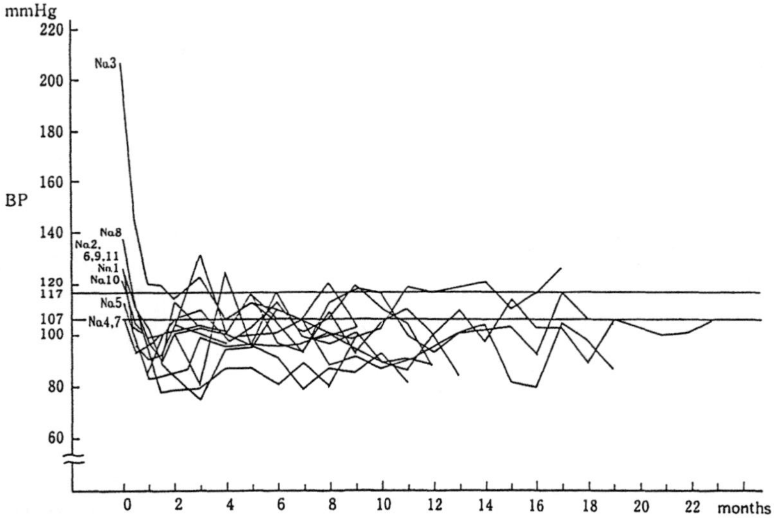

Fig. 2. Changes in mean blood pressure for all hypertensive patients during treatment with nifedipine tablet

Table 2. Changes in blood pressure

Blod pressure (mm Hg)	Marked ($n=8$)	Moderate ($n=1$)		Slight ($n=1$)		No unchange ($n=1$)	
Systolic	<-30	$-29<$	<-20	$-19<$	<-10	$-9<$	$<+9$
Diastolic	<-15	$-14<$	<-10	$-9<$	<-5	$-4<$	$<+4$
Mean	<-20	$-19<$	<-13	$-12<$	<-7	$-6<$	$<+6$

No significant change in heart rate was observed during the study except for only one point at 2 months after the treatment with nifedipine tablet (Fig. 3). Adverse effects were reported from three patients. Dizziness in two cases disappeared within a few days, and flashes with dizziness in one case required ceasing antihypertensive treatment because blood pressure levels of this patient fell to about 100/70 mmHg.

Values for laboratory examinations before and 6 months after treatment with nifedipine tablet are shown in Table 3. The data presented here were obtained exactly 6 months after the initiation of the study. Not all the patients, therefore, were subjected to these laboratory examinations, however, we could not determine any abnormal changes in laboratory data for the parameters examined. Several weeks before and after the point of 6 months, laboratory examinations were performed for the remaining patients, and none showed significant changes in any parameters directly related to administration of nifedipine tablet.

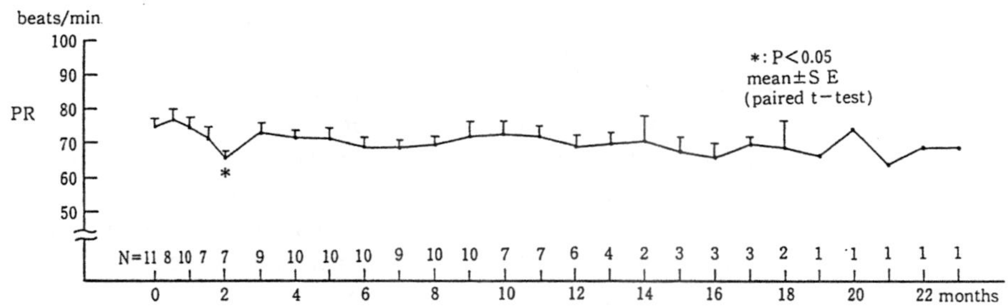

Fig. 3. Changes in heart rate during treatment with nifedipine tablet in essential and renal hypertensive patients

Table 3. Changes in values for laboratory examinations

Parameter	*n*	Before	After
RBC ($\times 10^4$/mm^3)	7	441.6±90.0	453.0±103.9
Hb (g/dl)	7	14.2±2.9	14.3±3.4
Ht (%)	7	41.0±8.0	42.5±9.9
WBC ($\times 10^2$/mm^3)	7	55.4±14.5	56.3±8.8
Platelet ($\times 10^4$/mm^3)	4	240.0±14.1	227.5±35.9
BUN (mg/dl)	6	23.0±9.5	28.0±21.6
Creatinine (mg/dl)	6	1.8±1.3	2.4±2.5
GOT (U)	8	16.1±2.9	20.0±3.9
GPT (U)	8	14.3±8.7	15.6±5.0
Al-p (KAU)	3	5.9±1.2	5.4±0.1
Al-p (IU)	2	54.5±3.5	64.0±11.3
LDH (U)	8	345.5±42.1	374.3±83.1
Uric acid (mg/dl)	6	6.2±1.6	6.2±1.0
Total cholesterol (mg/dl)	7	199.4±39.2	223.1±37.3
Na (mEq/l)	7	142.7±2.8	140.0±3.6
K (mEq/l)	7	4.2±0.5	4.2±0.9
Cl (mEq/l)	7	105.0±2.9	102.6±3.0
Ca (mg/dl)	7	9.6±0.2	9.6±1.2
P (mg/dl)	4	3.7±0.9	4.0±1.7
FBS (mg/dl)	3	96.7±15.8	91.0±6.6

Discussion

The aim of antihypertensive treatment for hypertensive patients is to minimize the organ damage due to sustained high blood pressure. Calcium antagonists such as nifedipine have been demonstrated to dilate vascular smooth muscle by inhibiting the inward current of calcium ion [4] which results in lowering blood pressure. Nifedipine, one of the dihydropyridine derivatives, has been reported to act on vascular muscle more selectively than cardiac muscle as compared to nondihydropyridine derivatives [5]. The original form of nifedipine in organic solvent has potent vasodilatory action with rapid onset [1]. The duration of action, however, is only about 4–6 h [2], which is not sufficiently long for use as an antihypertensive drug. To overcome this disadvantage, a retard form of nifedipine, nifedipine tablet, was developed. The antihypertensive effect of nifedipine tablet has been established to last more than 10–12 h in our hypertensive clinic (data not shown), which enables us to control high blood pressure by giving it twice daily.

In the present study, we have confirmed that nifedipine tablet is very effective in lowering blood pressure for a long period, not only in essential hypertensive patients but also in renal hypertensive subjects, by administering it twice daily with a dose range of 20–60 mg. In the case of nifedipine capsule the hypotensive effect was often accompanied with a reflex increase in heart rate [3], but this was not the case with nifedipine tablet in the current study. This may be explained at least in part by the fact that several patients included in this study had previously been treated with β-blockers or sympatholytic drugs. However, a somewhat smaller fluctuation in blood pressure is to be expected by treatment with nifedipine tablet than with nifedipine capsule, which may to some extent explain the lack of reflex tachycardia in the present study.

Because of its potent vasodilatory effect, nifedipine sometimes causes dizziness and flashes in patients. In the present study, 3 cases out of 11 complained of dizziness of flashes, but only one case required ceasing administration of nifedipine tablet because blood pressure had reached too low levels. No adverse effect on results from laboratory examinations was observed during the treatment with nifedipine tablet.

From these results, we concluded that nifedipine tablet administered twice daily is a useful antihypertensive drug for treatment of hypertensive patients without the risk of serious side effect.

References

1. Hashimoto K, Taira N, Chiba S, Hashimoto K jr, Endoh M, Kokubun M, Kokubun H, Iijima T, Kimura T, Kubota K, Oguro K (1972) Cardiohemodynamic effects of Bay a 1040 in the dog. Arzneimittelforschung 22:15–21
2. Hiwatari M, Satoh K, Taira N (1979) Antihypertensive effect of nifedipine on conscious renal-hypertensive dogs. Arzneimittelforschung 29:256–260
3. Imai Y, Abe K, Otsuka Y, Irokawa N, Yasujima M, Sato K, Sakurai Y, Chiba S, Ito T, Sato M, Haruyama T, Miura Y, Yoshinaga K (1980) Management of severe hypertension with nifedipine in combination with clonidine or propranolol. Arzneimittelforschung 30:674–678
4. Fleckenstein A (1981) Fundamental actions of calcium antagonists on myocardial and cardiac pacemaker cell membranes. In: Weiss GB (ed) New perspectives on calcium antagonists. American Physiological Society, Bethesda, pp 59–81
5. Himori N, Ono H, Taira N (1976) Simultaneous assessment of effects of coronary vasodilators on the coronary blood flow and myocardial contractility by using the blood-perfused canine papillary muscle. Jpn J Pharmacol 26:427–435

Hemodynamic and Neurohumoral Effects of Nifedipine Slow-Release Tablet in the Treatment of Hypertension

T. Santoso[1], D. Ismail[1], A. M. Rahman[1], M. N. T. Wangge[1], H. Mansjoer[1], T. Sugiarti[1], and N. Abdurahman[1]

Introduction

Nifedipine has been found effective in the acute [1–7] and long-term treatment [8–12] of hypertension. Hemodynamically the drug acts as a powerful arterial vasodilator [8, 13, 14] leading to a reduction in the elevated peripheral vascular resistance which is the hallmark of the established phase of essential hypertension [14, 15]. Following oral administration similar bioavailability was found for the various oral forms: 10-mg quick-release capsules or tablets and the 20-mg slow-release tablets. Plasma half-life for the standard capsule or tablet formulation is only 2.5–5 h. On the other hand, a very long half-life of 12–15 h may be observed after the administration of the retard tablets [16], making them theoretically more suitable for the long-term treatment of hypertension than the other oral nifedipine preparations.

The purpose of this study was to evaluate the effects of nifedipine slow-release tablets on blood pressure, heart rate, hemodynamics as assessed echocardiographically, plasma renin activity, and plasma catecholamines in patients with mild to moderate essential hypertension.

Methods

Patients: Nineteen asymptomatic ambulatory hypertensive patients (ten men and nine women) gave their informed consent to the study. Their ages ranged from 30 to 61 years (mean, 50 years). All patients had a supine diastolic blood pressure between 90 and 114 mmHg after a 2-week placebo run-in period. Causes of secondary hypertension were excluded by routine investigations. Excluded were patients with severe arrhythmia, angina pectoris, clinical symptoms of heart failure, pregnant women and women of child-bearing potential without adequate contraception, malignancies, psychoses, infections, severe diseases of the liver and/or kidney (serum creatinine 2.0 mg/dl or more), diabetes mellitus, or anemia and all patients for whom participation in

[1] Department of Internal Medicine, University of Indonesia, Medical School, Jakarta, Indonesia

the study would entail unacceptable risk to their health. As hemodynamic evaluation was performed by echocardiography, the patients were also selected on the basis of good-quality echocardiograms and the absence of regional wall motion abnormality on two-dimensional echocardiography.

Study Design: Patients were given placebo tablets twice daily for 2 weeks. Then they were randomized into a double-blind, cross-over trial of two 3-week periods during which they received twice daily 20-mg nifedipine slow-release tablets or placebo. The placebo wash-out period was 1 week (Fig. 1). No other medications were allowed during the study period; sodium intake was not controlled. Patient examinations were performed in the morning in an air-conditioned room after 30 min rest in recumbent position. All patients were requested to refrain from tobacco, tea, and caffeinated beverages for at least 12 h prior to study to avoid unwanted stimulation of sympathetic activity [17, 18]. Blood pressure and electrocardiographic examinations were made in weekly intervals. Echocardiographic recordings and determinations of plasma renin activity and plasma noradrenalin were performed at the beginning and in the last days of the placebo and treatment periods. All examinations were carried out 2 h 4 h after the morning dose has been taken.

Blood Pressure and Heart Rate Measurements: Right arm blood pressure measurements in the supine and standing positions were taken three times using cuff sphygmomanometer, and their average was reported. K1 and K4 were used for systolic (P_{syst}) and diastolic pressure (P_{diast}) determinations, respectively. Mean blood pressure (MBP) was calculated using the formula: $MBP = (P_{syst} + 2\ P_{diast})/3$. Heart rate (HR) was determined from an average of five RR intervals on the electrocardiographic recordings.

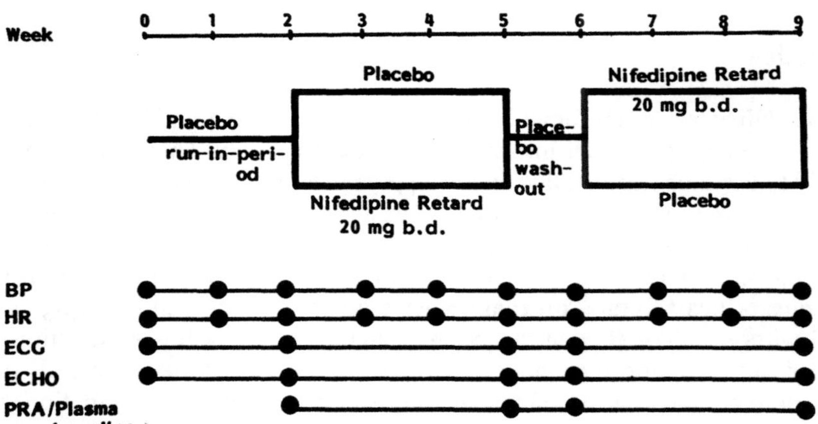

Fig. 1. Design of trial. *BP,* Blood pressure; *HR,* heart rate; *PRA,* plasma renin activity; *PNA,* plasma noradrenaline

Echocardiographic and Hemodynamic Measurements: Echocardiographic examinations were performed with the patient in the left lateral decubitus position. Left ventricular end-diastolic and -systolic dimensions (LVEDD, LVESD) were measured following recommendations of the Joint International Society and Federation of Cardiology/World Health Organization task force on recommendations for standardization of measurements from M-mode echocardiograms [19].

The following parameters were calculated:

- Fractional shortening (FS) = (LVEDD – LVESD)/LVEDD
- Cardiac output (CO) = stroke volume (SV) × HR, where SV was determined using Teichholtz' formula [20]
- Systemic vascular resistance (SVR) = Co/MBP × 80
- Wall thickness index (WTI) = 1/2 (IVS + PW), where PW is posterior wall thickness, and IVS is interventricular septal wall thickness
- Wall stress index (WSI) [21]:
  At end diastole: $WSI_{ed} = 0.5\ (P_{syst}\ LVEDD)/WTI$ at end diastole
  At end systole: $WSI_{es} = 0.5\ (P_{syst}\ LVESD)/WTI$ at end systole
- Left ventricular mass (LVM) [22]: LVM = 1.04 [(LVEDD + PW + IVS) – (LVID)] – 14 g

Plasma Assay: Plasma renin activity was measured by radioimmunoassay using Phadebas Angiotensin I Test (OY Medix AB, Finland). Plasma noradrenalin was measured by ^{3}H-labeled radioenzymatic assay (Amersham, UK).

Statistical Analysis: The paired Student's *t* test was used to analyze the significance of differenses between group means. Correlation coefficients were calculated to determine the relationship between percent change in PBP, baseline and change in plasma renin activity, and change in plasma noradrenaline.

Results

Effects on Blood Pressure and Heart Rate: Nifedipine slow-release tablet reduced supine P_{syst} and P_{diast} by 18.4% and 14.1%, respectively ($p<0.001$), and standing P_{syst} and P_{diast} by 21.1% and 17.4% ($p<0.001$). No orthostatic hypotension was noted. HR did not change (Table 1). In 14 patients (74%) a target blood pressure of 160/90 mmHg was achieved.

Effects on Echocardiographic and Hemodynamic Parameters: Nifedipine slow-release tablet significantly decreased the LVESD (–12.2%; $p<0.01$) and increased the fractional chortening (+24.2%; $p<0.001$), SV (+18.1%; $p<0.001$), and CO (+18.3%; $p<0.001$). SVR fell to 24.3% lower than in the pretreatment period ($p<0.001$). A reduction in WSI_{ed} (–14.9%) and WSI_{es} (–28.1%) ($p<0.001$) was also observed. LVEDD, WTI, and LVM did not change (Table 1).

Table 1. Effects of nifedipine slow-release tablet and placebo administration on blood pressure, heart rate, and echocardiographic-hemodynamic parameters

	Placebo		Nifedipine	
	Before	After	Before	After
BP (mm Hg)				
Supine				
P_{syst}	169±12	172±14	174±11	142±12[b]
P_{diast}	102±9	106±12	106±10	91±10[b]
Standing				
P_{syst}	170±12	172±14	175±10	138±11[b]
P_{diast}	108± 9	109±11	109± 9	90±10[b]
HR (beats/min)	74±10	75±10	80±11	80±10
LVEDD (mm)	48.7±4.8	48.7±5.4	48.8±4.1	48.6±4.3
LVESD (mm)	30.2±5.1	31.5±5.2	32.9±5.1	28.9±5.2[a]
FS (%)	38.0±6.1	35.3±5.4	32.5±5.0	40.3±5.3[b]
SV (ml)	72.7±13.8	70.3±12.5	67.5±13.7	79.7±13.4[b]
CO (l/min)	5.38±1.37	5.29±1.37	5.40±1.00	6.39±2.20[b]
SVR (dsc-5)	1980±600	2093±694	1965±449	1487±510[b]
WTI_{ed}	10.8±2.0	10.6±1.4	11.3±1.6	11.2±2.0
WSI_{ed}	375±76	374±51	377±52	321±53[b]
WSI_{es}	182±52	193±47	203±49	146±51[b]
LVM (g)	236±95	230±91	252±67	243±79

[a] $p<0.01$ [b] $p<0.001$

Effect on Neurohumoral Substances: The antihypertensive effect of nifedipine slow-release tablet correlated inversely with baseline plasma renin activity (Fig. 2). There was, however, no change in plasma renin activity or plasma noradrenalin resulting from the fall in blood pressure (Figs. 3, 4).

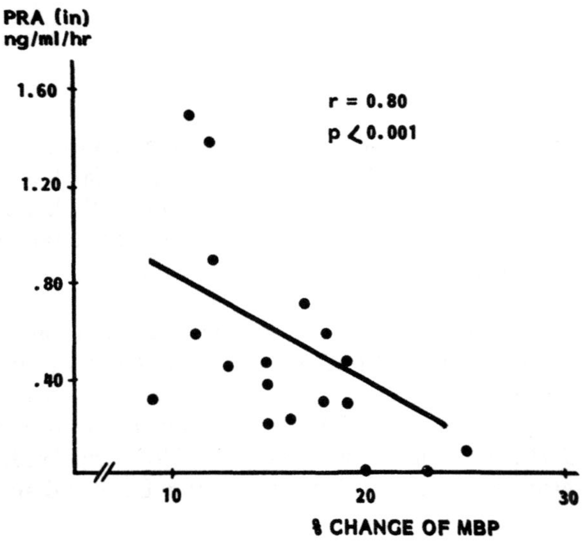

Fig. 2. Relation between baseline plasma renin activity and antihypertensive effect of nifedipine slow-release tablet. *MBP,* Mean blood pressure; *PRA,* plasma renin activity

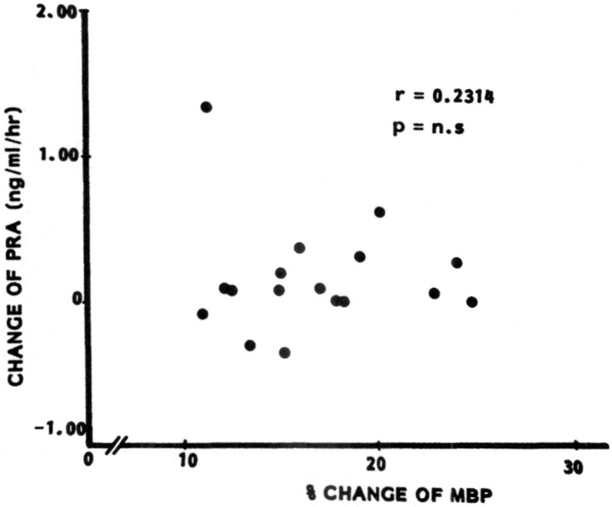

Fig. 3. Relation between change in plasma renin activity and fall in blood pressure

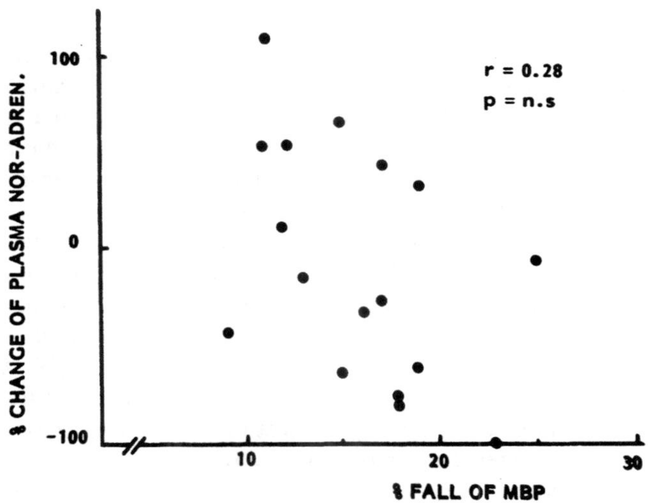

Fig. 4. Relation between change in plasma noradrenaline and fall in blood pressure

Side Effects: Side effects reported during nifedipine treatment were headache (two patients), flushing (one patient), and ankle edema (one patient). One patient reported headache while he was on placebo treatment.

Discussion

There has been a trend away from the view that nifedipine is not indicated for the treatment of mild hypertension [23], and clinical data are accumulating rapidly supporting the view that the drug may be useful in all grades of hypertension [24]. Nifedipine slow-release tablet (Adalat Retard) contains a crystalline form of nifedipine which delays absorption. This means that the fall in blood pressure occurs more slowly, particularly with the first dose [16, 25]. Since the half-life is 12–15 h, the drug is expected to possess a longer duration of antihypertensive action than the quick-release capsules or tablet form [16]. Although one study failed to show satisfactory results [26], other trials suggested that this preparation is effective for the long-term treatment of mild to moderate hypertension [27, 28]. We have confirmed this finding in our medium-term study.

The blood pressure fall was accompanied by a decrease in SVR indicating that this effect is mediated primarily through peripheral arteriolar dilatation [8, 13, 14]. The absence of orthostatic hypotension suggests that significant peripheral venodilatation is unlikely. Resetting of baroreceptor, which has been observed during chronic therapy [29], is also perhaps beneficial in preventing the orthostatic hypotension experienced by patients treated with other vasodilators.

Acutely, the decrease in systemic vascular resistance after nifedipine administration, especially in the capsule form, may cause transient activation of the sympathetic tone, which results in parallel increases in HR, indices of left ventricular contractility, CO, and plasma noradrenalin concentrations [3, 8–16]. Changes in MBP correlate inversely with the arterial baroreflex sensitivity, suggesting that arterial baroreflex mechanisms by means of sympathetic activation tend to limit the acute antihypertensive response [29]. This reflex may be avoided by slow rates of drug input [3], which may include giving the drug with food [30] or using the slow-release preparation to delay its absorption. With longer term administration, blood pressure but not SVR may decrease further as compared with the acute effect [29]. Chronically, there was also no significant change in HR and plasma noradrenalin level in this and other studies [9, 29–31], indicating a return toward control values of the acutely increased sympathetic activity. This phenomenon seems to play an important role in the further decrease in blood pressure during long-term nifedipine administration. And, indeed, an inverse relation between chronic changes in HR and in blood pressure was reported [29].

Although indices of left ventricular contractility usually tend to return toward pretreatment values, an increase in CO and FS measured noninvasively using echocardiography and cardiac inex measured by dye dilution technique may still be observed [23, 29, 32]. Likewise, we still found a mild increase in FS, SV, and CO after 3 weeks treatment. There are obviously some limitations in the assessment of left ventricular contractility indices from echocardiography, however the method has been found to produce values that correlate with those obtained invasively [20]. In addition, two-dimensional echocardiography in multiple views did not demonstrate asynergy in all patients, and these also serve as their own controls. Therefore, the relative changes in measured echocardiographic-hemodynamic parameters, if not the absolute values, should be reliable in this study [33–35]. Some degree of sympathetic activity may also persist on a long-term basis, however this is more likely to occur in nonresponders [29]. The mechanism of changes reflected in the increased left ventricular contractility indices should therefore be attributed to factors other than sympathetic overactivity, such as a decreased afterload [23, 36, 37] or improved abnormal diastolic function in hypertensive patients [38–40].

Since long-standing hypertension, particularly in the elderly, is often characterized not only by increased peripheral vascular resistance but also by a reduced CO nifedipine should therefore represent a logical therapeutic approach in such conditions [41, 42]. The decrease in blood pressure is not accompanied by an increase in HR resulting in a fall in the HR-pressure product, which is a major determinant of cardiac work. The WSI reflects the major determinant of the degree of left ventricular hypertrophy and plays a predominant role in both left ventricular function and myocardial energy balance [43]. The decrease in WSI may therefore be beneficial in the prevention and treatment of hypertensive heart disease. The short observations period, however, did not allow us to document any significant change in LVM. In general, reduction of LVM becomes evident after 8–12 weeks of antihypertensive therapy [44].

Most studies have reported a rise in plasma renin activity after acute nifedipine administration to healthy volunteers or patients with hypertension [2, 9, 16, 23, 24, 31]. This rise in renin is associated with an increse in sympathetic tone as judged by an increase in plasma noradrenalin [31]. Other factors may also be implicated, such as the loss of sodium that occurs with nifedipine and a direct effect of nifedipine on calcium transport across the macula densa [45]. With more chronic therapy, the increase in renin release is usually less conspicuous [9, 31, 46, 47]. This discrepancy in the effect of the drug on plasma renin activity during acute and long-term treatment is often ascribed to a diminishing sympathetic tone in the long term. This concept is also supported by our data. It has also been observed that the rise in plasma renin activity after acute nifedipine administration can be abolished by β-adrenoceptor blockade [46, 48]. The higher antihypertensive effect of nifedipine in patients with lower plasma renin activity found in the present study has confirmed the previous observations of Bühler et al. [49].

The low incidence of side effects may be related to the smoother, long-duration action of the slow-release preparation. It is noteworthy that patients who can not tolerate the capsule form may have no complaints while on the slow-release drug [50].

Acknowledgements: We express our deepest appreciation to R. Taruli, MD, for his help in data collecting, to Dr. Med. Thomas Korompis and Dr. Dr. Jap Tjiang Beng from Bayer for their support, to Dra. Endang Hoyaranda and her staff members from Prodia Laboratory for all their kind efforts and the careful laboratory investigations, and to Mrs. Tati Hidayat for preparation of the manuscript.

References

1. Guazzi MD, Olivari MT, Polese A, Fiorentini C, Magrini F, Moruzzi P (1977) Nifedipine, a new antihypertensive agent with rapid action. Clin Pharmacol Ther 22:528-532
2. Aoki K, Kondo S, Mochizuki A, Yoshida T, Kato S, Kato K, Takikawa K (1978) Antihypertensive effects of cardiovascular Ca^{2+} antagonist in hypertension patients in the absence and presence of beta-adrenergic-blockade. Am Heart J 96:218-226
3. Lederballe Pedersen O, Mikkelsen E (1978) Acute and chronic effects of nifedipine in arterial hypertension. Eur J Clin Pharmacol 14:375-381
4. Beer N, Gallegos I, Cohen A, Klein N, Sonnenblick E, Frishman W (1981) Efficacy of sublingual nifedipine in the acute treatment of systemic hypertension. Chest 79:571-574
5. Huysmans FTM, Thien TA, Sluiter HE, Koene RAP (1983) Acute treatment of hypertension with nifedipine. Neth J Med 26:256-261
6. Bertel O, Conen D, Radve EW, Muller J, Lang C, Dubach VC (1983) Nifedipine in hypertensive emergencies. Br Med J 286:19-20
7. Haft JI, Litterer WE (1984) Chewing nifedipine to rapidly treat hypertension. Arch Intern Med 144:2347-2359
8. Olivari MT, Bartorelli C, Polese A, Fiorentini C, Moruzzi P, Guazzi M (1979) Treatment of hypertension with nifedipine, a calcium antagonist agent. Circulation 59:1056-1062
9. Corea L, Miele M, Bentivoglio E, Boschetti E, Agabiti-Rosei E, Muiesan G (1979) Acute and chronic effects of nifedipine in plasma renin activity and plasma adrenaline and noradrenaline in controls and hypertensive patients. Clin Sci 57:115s-117s
10. Maeda K, Tanaka C, Tsukano Y, Minamikawa H, Komatsu H, Kotsumi K, Inoue E (1982) Antihypertensive effects of the calcium antagonist agent nifedipine. Arzneimittelforschung 32:267-271
11. Litter WA, Stallard TJ, Watson RDS, McLeay RAB (1983) The effect of nifedipine on arterial blood pressure and reflex cardiac control. Postgrad Med J 59 [Suppl 2]:109-113
12. Masotti G, Pogessi L, Castellani S, Morettini A, Galanti G, Scarti L (1984) A study of the antihypertensive effect and some pharmacodynamic aspects of nifedipine in medium-term treatment. In J Clin Pharmacol Res 4:71-79
13. Lund-Johansen P, Omvik P (1983) Hemodynamic effects of nifedipine in essential hypertension at rest and during exercise. J Hypertens 1:159-163
14. Lund-Johansen P (1985) Hemodynamic effects of calcium channel blockers at rest and during exercise in essential hypertension. Am J Med 79 [Supp 4A]:11-18
15. Lund-Johansen P (1980) State of the art review: hemodynamics in essential hypertension. Clin Sci 59:343s-354s
16. Kuhlman J, Graeffe KH, Pämsch KD, Ziegler R (1986) Clinical pharmacology. In: Krebs R (ed) Treatment of cardiovascular diseases by Adalat (nifedipine). Schattauer, Stuttgart, pp 93-144
17. Cryer PE, Haymond MV, Santiago JV, Shah SD (1976) Norepinephrine and epinephrine release and adrenergic mediation of smoking-associated hemodynamic and metabolic events. N Engl J Med 295:573-577
18. Robertson D, Fröhlich JC, Carr RK (1978) Effects of caffeine on plasma renin activity, catecholamines, and blood pressure. N Engl J Med 298:181-184
19. O'Rourke RA, Hanrath P, Henry WN, Hugenholtz PG, Pisa Z, Roelandt J, Tanaka M (1984) Report of the Joint International Society and Federation of Cardiology/World

Health Organization. Task force on recommendation for standardization of measurements from M-mode echocardiograms. Circulation 69:854A–857A
20. Teichholz LE, Kreulen T, Herman MV, Gorlin R (1976) Problems in echocardiographic volume determinations: echocardiographic-angiographic correlations in the presence or absence of asynergy. Am J Cardiol 37:7–11
21. Quinones MA, MOkotoff DM, Nouri S, Winters WL jr, Miller RR (1980) Noninvasive quantification of left ventricular wall stress: validation of method and application to assessment of chronic pressure overload. Am J Cardiol 45:482–485
22. Devereux R, Reichek N (1977) Echocardiographic determination of left ventricular mass in man. Circulation 55:613–616
23. Guazzi MD, Polese A, Fiorentini C, Bartorell A, Moruzzi P (1983) Treatment of hypertension with calcium antagonist: review. Hypertension 5 [Suppl II]:85–90
24. Sorkin EM, Clissold SP, Brogden RN (1985) Nifedipine. A review of its pharmacodynamic and pharmacokinetic properties, and therapeutic efficacy, in ischaemic heart disease, hypertension and related cardiovascular disorders. Drugs 30:182–274
25. Taburet AM. Singlas E, Colin JN, Banzet O, Thibonnier M, Corvol P (1983) Pharmacokinetic studies of nifedipine tablet correlation with antihypertensive effects. Hypertension 5:II29–II33
26. Brennan FN, Blake S (1982) The use of nifedipine as a third-step agent in the treatment of refractory hypertension. Ir Med J 75:29–30
27. Englert R (1984) Verlaufsbeobachtungen über 2 Jahre bei Hypertoniepatienten mit Adalat-retard. Wien Med Wochenschr 134 [Suppl 82]:7–8
28. Landmark K (1985) Antihypertensive and metabolic effects of long term therapy with nifedipine slow release tablets. J Cardiovasc Pharmacol 7:12–17
29. Kiowski W, Erne P, Bertel O, Bolli, Bühler F (1986) Acute and chronic sympathetic reflex activation and antihypertensive response to nifedipine. J Am Coll Cardiol 7:344–348
30. Hirasawa K, Shen WF, Kelly DT, Roubin G, Tateda K, Shibata J (1985) Effect of food investigation on nifedipine absorption and haemodynamic response. Eur J Clin Pharmacol 28:105–107
31. Lederballe Pederson O, Mikkelsen E, Christensen NJ, Kornerup HJ, Pedersen EB (1979) Effect of nifedipine on plasma renin, aldosterone and catecholamines in arterial hypertension. Eur J Clin Pharmacol 15:235–240
32. Landmark K, Dale J (1985) Antihypertensive, hemodynamic and metabolic effects of nifedipine slow-release tablets in elderly patients. Acta Med Scand 218:389–396
33. Reichek N (1987) Standardization in the measurement of left ventricular mass. M mode echocardiography. Hypertension 9 [Supp 2 pt 2]:II 27–29
34. Wallerson DC, DEvereux RB (1987) Reproducibility of echocardiographic left ventricular measurements. Hypertension 9 [Suppl 2 pt 2]:II 6–18
35. Devereux RB (1987) Detection of left ventricular hypertrophy by M-mode echocardiography. Anatomic validation, standardization, and comparison to other methods. Hypertension 9 [Suppl 2 pt 2]:II9–26
36. Kurnik PB, Tiefenbrunn AJ, Ludbrook PA (1984) The dependence of the cardiac effects of nifedipine on the responses of the peripheral vascular system. Circulation 69:963–972
37. Ludbrook PA, Tiefenbrunn AJ, Reed FR, Sobel BE (1982) Acute hemodynamic responses to sublingual nifedipine: dependence on left ventricular function. Circulation 65:489–498
38. Polese A, Fiorentini C, Olivari MT, Guazzi MD (1979) Clinical use of a calcium antagonistic agent (nifedipine) in acute pulmonary edema. Am J Med 66:825–830
39. Ratts TE, Addington B, Gerlach P, Conway L, Sullivan JM (1984) Left ventricular function in heart failure and hypertension: an echocardiographic-clinical study. In: 10th scientific meeting, international society of hypertension, Interlaken, June 17–21, p 727
40. Rosanelli G, Agabiti-Rosei E, Mueisan M (1984) Systeolic and diastolic ventricular function in essential hypertension as related to left ventricular mass and adrenergic ac-

tivity. In: 10th scientific meeting, international society of hypertension, Interlaken, June 17–21, p 742

41. Messerli FH, Venture HO, Glade LB, Sundgaard-Riise K, Dunn FG, Fröhlich ED (1983) Essential hypertension in the elderly: hemodynamics, intravascular volume, plasma renin activity and circulating catecholamine levels. Lancet ii:983–986
42. Kaplan NM (1982) Clinical hypertension, 3rd edn. Williams and Wilkins, Baltimore, pp 42–97
43. Strauer BE (1981) Performance, wall dynamics and coronary function of the left ventricle in hypertensive heart disease. In: Strauer BE (ed) The heart in hypertension. Springer, Berlin Heidelberg New York, pp 251–284
44. Fouad-Tarazi FM, Liebson PR (1987) Echocardiographic studies of regression of left ventricular hypertrophy in hypertension. Hypertension 9 [Supp 2 pt 2]: II 65–68
45. MacGregor GA (1986) Hypertension. In: Krebs R (ed) Treatment of cardiovascular diseases by Adalat (nifedipine). Schattauer, Stuttgart pp 231–258
46. Corea L, Alunni G, Bentivoglio M, Boschetti E, Cosmi F et al. (1980) Acute and long term effects of nifedipine on plasma catecholamines in controls and hypertensive patients before and after metoprolol. Acta Therapeut 6:177–187
47. Kiowski W, Bertel O, Erne P, Bolli P, Hulthen L et al. (1983) Hemodynamic and reflex responses to acute and chronic antihypertensive therapy responses to acute and chronic antihypertensive therapy with the calcium entry blocker nifedipine. Hypertension 5 [Suppl I]:70–74
48. Ekelund LG, Ekelund C, Rössner S (1982) Antihypertensive effects at rest and during exercise of a calcium blocker, nifedipine, alone and in combination with metroprolol. Acta Med Scan 212:71–75
49. Bühler FR, Hulthen UL, Kiowski W, Bolli P (1983) β-Blockers and calcium antagonists: cornerstones of antihypertensive therapy in the 1980. Drugs 25 [Suppl 2]:50–57
50. Bursztyn M, Grossmann E, Rosenthal T (1984) Long acting nifedipine in the treatment of severe hypertension. Eur J Clin Pharmacol 27:13–17

Special Topics

Effect of Nifedipine on Serum Lipoprotein Metabolism in Patients with Essential Hypertension

K. Arakawa[1] and J. Sasaki[1]

Introduction

Nifedipine is a calcium channel blocker that has been widely used for the treatment of hypertension (Olivari et al. 1979) and coronary artery disease (Henry 1980; Hugenholtz et al. 1981). Some antihypertensive agents have been shown to influence lipoprotein concentrations (Weidmann et al. 1985). Although some controversial data have been reported, prolonged use of chlorothiazide increases serum total cholesterol and serum triglyceride levels (Weidmann et al. 1985). β-Blockers increase triglyceride and decrease high-density lipoprotein cholesterol (HDL-C) levels (Weidmann et al. 1985). On the other hand, α_1-blockers decrease total cholesterol and triglyceride levels and increase HDL-C and the ratio of HDL to low-density liproprotein (Weidmann et al. 1985). However, the effect of calcium channel blockers on lipoprotein metabolism is unclear. Several studies showed no significant change in total cholesterol, triglyceride, and HDL-C with nifedipine (Pasanisi et al. 1986; Vessby et al. 1983; Weidmann et al. 1985) and verapamil (Faergeman et al. 1982; Lewis 1986; Walldius 1982) whereas others reported increased HDL-C with diltiazem (Pool et al. 1985) and nicardipine (Ishida et al. 1984).

In the present study, we have measured, serum lipids and lipoproteins including the HDL subfractions HDL_2-C and HDL_3-C, which are important factors in atherogenesis, following the administration of nifedipine to patients with mild essential hypertension.

Subjects and Methods

A total of 45 patients with mild essential hypertension (systolic blood pressure over 160 mmHg and/or diastolic blood pressure over 95 mmHg) were included in the study. The age of patients ranged from 31 to 76 years (mean, 59.8 years). There were 18 men and 27 women. None of the patients had major complications such as ischemic heart disease, stroke, renal disease, or

[1] Department of Internal Medicine, Fukuoka University Hospital, Fukuoka, Japan

hepatic disease. Cases with secondary hypertension were excluded. None of the drugs which are known to affect lipid concentrations was given. Informed consent was obtained from patients before the study. After a washout period of 4 weeks, during which any antihypertensive drugs were withdrawn, patients were given 30 mg nifedipine per day (t.i.d.; $n=28$) or 40 mg nifedipine retard per day (b.i.d.; $n=17$) over a period of 16 weeks. All patients were asked to maintain their normal lifestyle regarding diet and exercise during the study.

Blood was drawn via venipuncture after at least 12 h fast. Cholesterol and triglyceride levels were quantitated enzymatically (Allain et al. 1974; Eggstein and Kreutz 1966). Lipoproteins were separated by ultracentrifugation with KBr for density adjustment (Havel et al. 1955). Statistical significance was evaluated using the paired Student's *t* test.

Results

Systolic and diastolic blood pressure decreased significantly after nifedipine (Fig. 1), and triglyceride decreased significantly after nifedipine (176±23 mg/

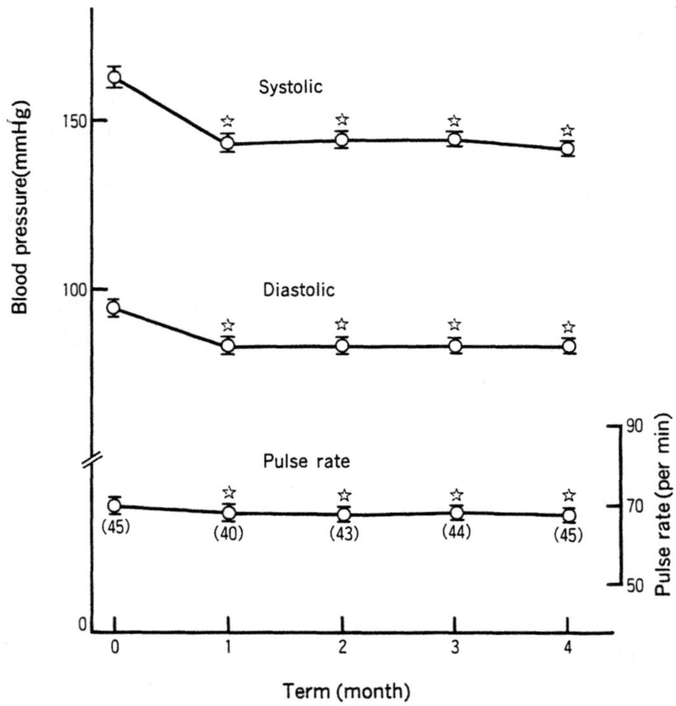

Fig. 1. Effect of nifedipine on blood pressure and pulse rate. *, $p<0.01$, compared with baseline value

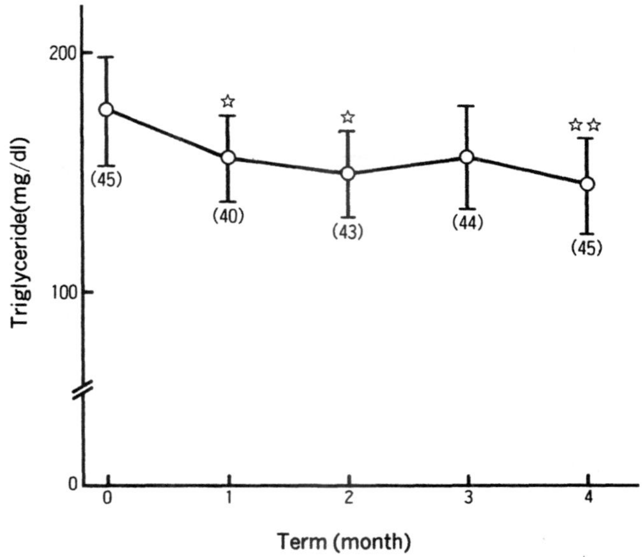

Fig. 2. Effect of nifedipine on serum triglyceride. *, $p<0.05$, compared with baseline value; **, $p<0.01$, compared with baseline value

dl before, 145±20 mg/dl after 4 months; Fig. 2). Total cholesterol and LDL-C did not change after nifedipine. HDL_2-C increased significantly (29.5±1.5 mg/dl before, 32.5±1.5 mg/dl after 4 months), and HDL_3-C decreased significantly (18.9±0.8 mg/dl before, 17.4±0.6 mg/dl after 4 months) after nifedipine (Fig. 3). No significant change was observed in total HDL-C after nifedipine. A significant increase in the HDL_2-C/HDL_3-C ratio (1.68±0.11 before, 2.01±0.13 after 4 months) was observed after nifedipine. No significant change was observed in the LDL-C/HDL-C ratio after nifedipine.

Discussion

In the present study, we observed after nifedipine a significant decrease in triglyceride, increase in HDL_2-C, decrease in HDL_3-C, and increase in the HDL_2-C/HDL_3-C ratio but no change in total HDL-C. Recently, Vessby et al. (1983) reported an increase in apolipoproteins A-I and A-II during nifedipine treatment in patients with essential hypertension, although no significant change was observed in total HDL-C. The influence of calcium channel blockers other than nifedipine on lipid metabolism has also been reported. Lewis (1986), Wallidus (1982), and Faergeman et al. (1982) reported that verapamil administration did not affect serum lipids and HDL-C, but Pool et al. (1985) showed increased HDL-C after diltiazem administration. Ishida et al. (1984) reported that treatment with nicardipine hydrochloride in patients

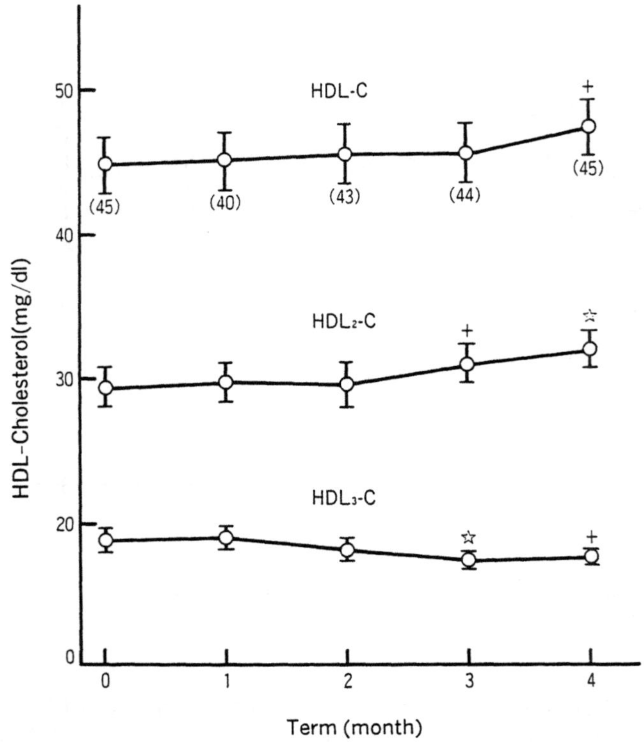

Fig. 3. Effect of nifedipine on serum high-density lipoprotein cholesterol *(HDL-C)*, HDL_2-C, and HDL_3-C. +, $p<0.1$, compared with baseline value. *, $p<0.05$, compared with baseline value

with hypertension, ischemic heart disease, and cerebrovascular disease increased HDL-C and decreased total cholesterol and triglyceride levels. Ohata et al. (1984) reported that nicardipine decreased LDL and increased HDL in rats. It has been well established that a low HDL level is a risk factor for coronary artery disease (Castelli et al. 1977; Gofman et al. 1966; Miller et al. 1977; Rhoads et al. 1976; Taskinen and Nikkila 1981), and the incidence of coronary artery disease is associated specifically with decreased HDL_2-C (Miller et al. 1977). Furthermore, Gofman et al. (1966) demonstrated that the HDL_2/HDL_3 ratio is lower in patients with than in patients without coronary artery disease. Therefore, the increased HDL_2-C and decreased HDL_2-C/HDL_3-C ratio presented in our study should be beneficial in decreasing the risk of ischemic heart disease.

The mechanism of increased HDL_2-C following administration of nifedipine remains unknown at present. Since the increase in HDL_2-C was associated with a significant decrease in triglyceride level following administration of nifedipine, increased catabolism of very low density lipoproteins probably via activation of lipoprotein lipase may contribute to this increase in

HDL_2-C. In addition, recent studies in rabbits (Henry and Bentley 1981) and on smooth muscle cells (Etingin and Hajjar 1984) have shown that nifedipine inhibits the formation of atherosclerotic lesions, although some studies have revealed no significant effect (Stender et al. 1984).

These findings suggest nifedipine to be a potential antiatherogenic drug. In view of the adverse effects of some antihypertensive drugs on lipid metabolism, nifedipine should be prefered in the treatment of hypertension.

References

Allain CC, Poon LS, Chan CS, Richmond W, Fu PC (1974) Enzymatic determination of total serum cholesterol. Clin Chem 20:470–475

CastelliWP, Doyle JT, Gordon T et al. (1977) HDL cholesterol and other lipids in coronary heart disease. The cooperative lipoprotein phenotyping study. Circulation 55:767–772

Eggstein M, Kreutz FH (1966) Eine neue Bestimmung der Neutralfette im Blutserum und Gewebe. I. Mitt. Prinzip, Durchführung und Besprechung der Methode. Klin Wochenschr 44:262–267

Etingin OR, Hajjar DP (1984) Nifedipine reduces cholesterol accumulation in lipid-laden arterial smooth muscle cells. Circulation 70 [Suppl]:II-138

Faergeman O, Meinerts H, Hansen F (1982) Serum lipoproteins after treatment with verapamil for 6 months. Acta Med Scand 681 [Suppl]:49–51

Gofman JW, Young W, Tandy R (1966) Ischemic heart disease, atherosclerosis and longevity. Circulation 34:679–697

Havel RJ, Edger HA, Bragdon JH (1955) The distribution and chemical composition of ultracentrifugally separated lipoproteins in human serum. J Clin Invest 34:1345–1353

Henry PD (1980) Comparative pharmacology of calcium antagonists: nifedipine, verapamil and diltiazem. Am J Cardiol 46:1047–1058

Henry PD, Bentley KI (1981) Suppression of atherogenesis in cholesterol-fed rabbit treated with nifedipine. J Clin Invest 68:1366–1369

Hugenholtz PG, Michels HR, Serruys PW, Brower PW (1981) Nifedipine in the treatment of unstable angina, coronary spasm and myocardial ischemia. Am J Cardiol 47:163–173

Ishida N, Matsuo R, Migita T, Tanaka Y, Fujimoto T, Baba Y, Inoue T, Satoh H, Satoh Y, Tohno T (1984) Effects of nicardipine HCl on serum lipids and blood pressure. J Jpn Atherosclerosis Soc 12:833–838 (with English abstr)

Lewis GRJ (1986) Long-term results with verapamil in essential hypertension and its influence on serum lipids. Am J Cardiol 57:35D–38D

Miller NE, Forde OH, Thelle DS et al. (1977) The Tromso heart study. High-density lipoprotein and coronary heart-disease: a prospective case control study. Lancet i:965–968

Ohata I, Sakamoto N, Nagano K, Maeno H (1984) Low density lipoprotein-lowering and high density lipoproteinelevating effects of nicardipine in rats. Biochem Pharmacol 33:2199–2205

Olivari MJ, Bartorelli C, Polese A, Fiorentini C, Moruzzi P, Guazzi MD (1979) Treatment of hypertension with nifedipine, a calcium antagonistic agent. Circulation 59:1059–1062

Pasanisi F, Ferrara AL, Lovine C, Mancini M (1986) Effects of nifedipine on insulin secretion and plasma lipids in hypertensive patients. Curr Ther Res Clin Exp 39:894–899

Pool PE, Seagren SC, Sable AF (1985) Effects of diltiazem on serum lipids, exercise performance and blood pressure: randomized, double-blind, placebo-controlled evaluation for systemic hypertension. Am J Cardiol 56:86H–91H

Rhoads, GG, Gulbrandsen CL, Kagan A (1976) Serum lipoproteins and coronary heart disease in a population study of Hawaii Japanese men. N Engl J Med 294:293–298

Stender S, Stender I, Nordestgaard B, Kjeldsen K (1984) No effect of nifedipine on atherogenesis in cholesterol-fed rabbit. Arteriosclerosis 4:389–394

Taskinen MR, Nikkila E (1981) High density lipoprotein subfractions in relation to lipoprotein lipase activety of tissues in man - evidence for reciprocal regulation of HDL_2 and HDL_3 levels by lipoprotein lipase. Clin Chim Acta 112:325–332
Vessby B, Abelin J, Finnson M, Hellsing K, Lithell H (1983) Effects of nifedipine treatment on carbohydrate and lipoprotein metabolism. Curr Ther Res Clin Exp 33:1075–1080
Walldius G (1982) Effect of verapamil on serum lipoproteins in patients with angina pectoris. Acta Med Scand 681 [Suppl]:43–48
Weidmann P. Uehlinger DE, Gerber A (1985) Antihypertensive treatment of serum lipoproteins. J Hypertens 3:297–306

Effects of Nifedipine on Cardiovascular System, with Special Reference to Coronary Circulation

Y. Hirota[1], G. Shimizu[1], K. Kaku[1], Y. Kita[1], T. Saito[1], and K. Kawamura[1]

Introduction

Hypertrophic cardiomyopathy (HCM) has been believed to be a disease of diastole, while systolic functions are normal or supernormal (Goodwin 1970; Wynne and Braunwald 1984). As such, the disease involves impaired left ventricular (LV) relaxation and reduced compliance. The traditional concept of supernormal systolic function has been questioned recently by some investigators (Hirota et al. 1982; Pouleur et al. 1983), and the development of congestive heart failure associated with dilated and poorly contracting left ventricle has received substantial attention (Fujiwara et al. 1984; Yutani et al. 1985; Fighali et al. 1987). Inadequate blood supply to the myocardium due either to elevated LV diastolic pressure or to the presence of small-vessel disease may be responsible for the clinical deterioration (Fujiwara et al. 1984; Maron et al. 1986).

Whereas β-blocking agents have been used in the treatment of HCM to reduce the outflow tract obstruction, nifedipine has recently been used to improve impaired diastolic function (Lorell et al.; Suwa et al. 1983).

We evaluated the effects of sublingually administered nifedipine on the cardiovascular system in patients with HCM during diagnostic cardiac catheterization, expecting this agent to have favorable effects on myocardial metabolism in addition to salutary effects on LV diastolic properties.

Methods

Six patients with HCM were the subjects of this study (Table 1). Their diagnoses were established according to the criteria of the WHO/ISFC recommendation (Brandenburg et al. 1981). All were males, aged from 18 to 55 years, and three had a family history of HCM. Echocardiographic examination revealed incomplete systolic anterior movement of the mitral valve in two of them. Four patients satisfied echocardiographic criteria of asymmetric

[1] Third Division, Department of Internal Medicine, Osaka Medical College, Takatsuki, Osaka, Japan

Table 1. Patient profiles

Case no.	Age (years)	Sex	FH	Echocardiogram			Cineangiogram		Blood level of nifedipine (ng/ml)
				IVS (mm)	PW (mm)	SAM	EDV (ml)	EF (%)	
1	55	M	–	(Poor record)			90	78	37.3
2	55	M	–	22	13	–	102	70	34.0
3	44	M	–	21	13	+	138	71	44.2
4	18	M	+	19	16	–	189	40	30.2
5	34	M	+	16	12	–	112	77	8.7
6	54	M	+	20	9	+	86	84	212.1

FH, Family history of hypertrophic cardiomyopathy; *IVS,* interventricular septum; *PW,* posterior wall; *SAM,* systolic anterior motion of the mitral valve; *EDV,* end-diastolic volume; *EF,* ejection fraction.

septal hypertrophy, and one had concentric LV hypertrophy. The LV free wall was thickest at the apex in one case (so-called apical hypertrophy; Yamaguchi et al. 1979). LV end-diastolic volume was in the normal range with normal or supernormal ejection fraction in five, and one had a dilated and poorly contracting left ventricle.

At the beginning of the diagnostic cardiac catheterization, an 8-F Mikro-tip angiocatheter was placed in the apical area of the left ventricle; a 7-F pigtail catheter in the ascending aorta; and 7-F Swan-Ganz and Webster catheters in the pulmonary artery and coronary sinus, respectively.

The measurements of intracardiac pressures, cardiac output, coronary sinus flow, and blood sampling from the ascending aorta and coronary sinus were performed initially. Nifedipine (Adalat) 10 mg was administered sublingually, and the same procedures were repeated 10–20 min after the administration. Blood samples were tested for oxygen content, lactate, pyruvate, and nifedipine concentrations. LV and coronary cineangiograms and biventricular endomyocardial biopsies were then performed in all cases. The paired Student's *t* test was applied for statistical analysis.

Results

Plasma levels ranged from 8.7 to 212.1 ng/ml at 20 min after the sublingual administration (Table 1). Hemodynamic data are presented in Tables 2 and 3. Heart rate was increased with nifedipine. LV systolic and end-diastolic pressures were decreased. Mean aortic, right atrial, and pulmonary arterial pressures did not change significantly. Cardiac output was increased probably due to the reduction in systemic vascular resistance, but no significant changes were observed in pulmonary arteriolar resistance. The index of contractility $(dP/dt)/DP_{40}$ was normal in all cases at rest (normal value of this laboratory, $32 \pm 7\ s^{-1}$; Hirota et al. 1982) and increased in all but one case.

Table 2. Hemodynamic changes with nifedipine in HCM

	HR (b/min)	MRAP (mm Hg)	LVEDP (mm Hg)	MPAP (mm Hg)	MAOP (mm Hg)	CO (l/min)	PAR (dynes·sec·cm^{-5})	SVR (dynes·sec·cm^{-5})	(dP/dt)/DP_{40} (sec^{-1})	T (ms)
Before	69±8	5±3	19±10	17±8	91±6	4.92±0.65	100±33	1450±230	33±6	85±25
After	78±9[a]	6±5	17± 9[b]	18±9	86±7	5.53±0.40[a]	120±54	1182±155[b]	35±5	77±23[b]

HR, Heart rate; *MRAP*, mean right atrial pressure; *LVEDP*, left ventricular end-diastolic pressure; *MPAP*, mean pulmonary artery pressure; *MAOP*, mean aortic pressure; *CO*, cardiac output; *PAR*, pulmonary arteriolar resistance; *SVR*, systemic vascular resistance; (dP/dt)/DP_{40}, dP/dt at developed pressure of 40 mm Hg divided by the developed pressure; *T*, time constant of the left ventricular pressure fall.

[a] $p<0.05$
[b] $p<0.01$

Table 3. Changes in coronary blood flow and resistance with nifedipine

	CSF (ml/min)	CAR (dynes · sec · cm^{-5})	MVO_2 (ml/min)	MLE (mg/min)
Before	139 ± 41	55 ± 23	14.0 ± 3.8	3.4 ± 1.9
After	164 ± 49[a]	43 ± 18[a]	14.5 ± 5.3	4.1 ± 1.8

CSF, Coronary sinus flow; *CAR,* coronary arteriolar resistance; *MVO_2,* myocardial oxygen consumption; *MLE,* myocardial lactate extraction.
[a] $p < 0.01$

The index of relaxation-time constant of LV pressure fall, was markedly prolonged before the administration and became shorter in all cases. These values were, however, still abnormally prolonged considering the normal value of 33 ± 8 ms (Hirota 1980).

Coronary blood flow was increased in all cases, with the reduction of calculated coronary arteriolar resistance. Myocardial oxygen consumption was increased in three, unchanged in one, and decreased in two cases. All patients had lactate extraction before nifedipine, and the extraction was increased in four of them after the administration. There was a linear relation between myocardial oxygen consumption and the double product of LV systolic pressure and heart rate with a high correlation coefficient ($r = 0.836$, $p < 0.001$; Fig. 1).

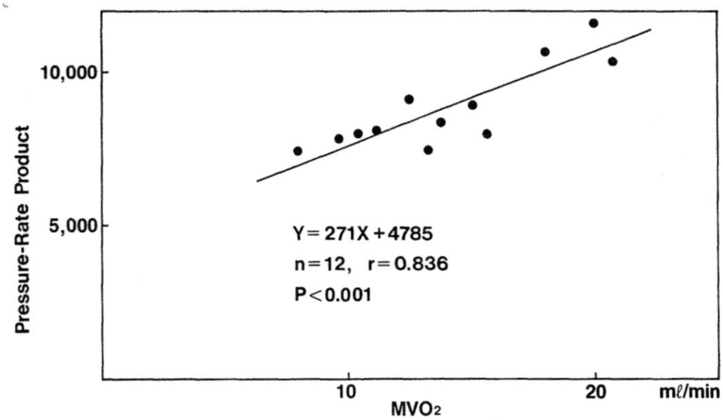

Fig. 1. Relationship between pressure-rate product and calculated myocardial oxygen consumption *(MVO_2)*. The correlation betweeen pressure-rate product and myocardial oxygen consumption was evaluated before and after nifedipine administration. The pressure-rate product is considered to be an indicator of myocardial oxygen demand. Actual oxygen consumption was calculated from the coronary sinus flow and aorto coronary sinus oxygen difference. This highly significant correlation suggested that changes of myocardial oxygen consumption with nifedipine is due to changes in demand

Discussion

Recent advances in the understanding of myocardial muscle mechanics and the natural history of HCM have changed the traditional concept of pathophysiological characteristics of this disease (Goodwin 1970; Wynne and Braunwald 1984), i.e., normal or supernormal systolic function and impaired diastolic properties. Hirota et al. (1982) and Pouleur and associated (1983) have proposed the possibility of depressed myocardial contractility by analysis of the force-length-velocity relationship. Several investigations have demonstrated that some patients develop congestive heart failure with the dilated and poorly contracting left ventricle, which is similar to that of dilated cardiomyopathy after long-term observations (Maron et al. 1979; Fujiwara et al. 1984;Yutani et al. 1985; Fighali et al. 1987). Either subendocardial ischemia due to inadequate blood supply with the elevated LV diastolic pressure or global ischemia and fibrosis because of small-vessel disease (Fujiwara et al. 1984; Maron et al. 1986) are thought to be the etiological factors.

Nifedipine has been used for the treatment of HCM since Lorell and associates (1982) reported that it can normalize the abnormal relaxation. Our data indicate abnormal LV isovolumic relaxation by the prolonged relaxation index in all six cases compared to the normal value of this laboratory (Hirota 1980). Although nifedipine improved abnormal isovolumic relaxation, it was not enough to normalize the prolonged relaxation index.

A potent arteriolar vasodilator, nifedipine has frequently been used for antihypertensive treatment and vasodilator therapy in patients with congestive heart failure. We have also demonstrated a potent arteriolar dilating effect in HCM. Therefore, nifedipine is the drug of choice in patients with HCM who have mild hypertension or somewhat deteriorated LV function.

Since inadequate coronary circulation has been emphasized, we evaluated the effect of nifedipine on coronary circulation and myocardial metabolism. All six patients had global aerobic metabolism before the administration of nifedipine as manifested by lactate consumption. Nifedipine was demonstrated to be a potent coronary arteriolar vasodilator and to increase coronary flow in HCM. Myocardial oxygen consumption and lactate extraction were increased in some, and decreased in others. The calculated myocardial oxygen consumption increased in some, and decreased in others. The calculated myocardial oxygen consumption was parallel to demand, showing a highly significant correlation to the pressure-rate product. Therefore, increased coronary blood flow by nifedipine seems to be due only to dilatation of the resistant vessel, and it is difficult to conclude from this investigation that nifedipine has salutary effects on myocardial metabolism and the oxygen delivery system.

References

Brandenburg RO, Chazov E, Cherian G, Falase AO, Grosgogeart Y et al. (1981) Report of the WHO/ISFC task force of definition and classification of cardiomyopathies. Circulation 64:437A–438A

Fighali S, Krajcer Z. Edelman S, Leachman RD (1987) Progression of hypertrophic cardiomyopathy into hypokinetic left ventricle: higher incidence in patients with midventricular obstruction. J Am Coll Cardiol 9:288–294

Fujiwara H, Onodera T, Tanaka M, Shirane H, Kato H et al. (1984) Progression from hypertrophic cardiomyopathy to typical dilated cardiomyopathy-like features in the end stage. Jpn Circ J 48:1210–1214

Goodwin JF (1970) Congestive and hypertrophic cardiomyopathy. A decade of study. Lancet i:731–739

Hirota Y (1980) A clinical study of left ventricular relaxation. Circulation 62:756–763

Hirota Y, Furubayashi K, Shimizu G, Kaku K, Kino M, Kawamura K, Takatsu T (1982) Hypertrophic nonobstructive cardiomyopathy: a precise assessment of hemodynamic characteristics and clinical implications. Am J Cardiol 50:990–997

Hirota Y, Shimizu G, Kaku K, Saito T, Kino M, Kawamura K (1984) Mechanisms of compensation and decompensation in dilated cardiomyopathy. Am J Cardiol 54:1033–1038

Lorell BH, Paulus WJ, Grossman W, Wynne J, Cohn PF (1982) Modification of abnormal left ventricular diastolic properties by nifedipine in patients with hypertrophic cardiomyopathy. Circulation 65:499–507

Maron BJ, Epstein SE, Roberts WC (1979) Hypertrophic cardiomyopathy and transmural myocardial infarction without significant atherosclerosis of the extramural coronary arteries. Am J Cardiol 43:1086–1102

Maron BJ, Wolfson JK, Epstein SE, Roberts WC (1986) Intramural ("small vessel") coronary artery disease in hypertrophic cardiomyopathy. J Am Coll Cardiol 8:545–557

Pouleur H, Rousseau MF, Eyll CV, Brasseur LA, Charlier AA (1983) Force-velocity-length relations in hypertrophic cardiomyopathy. Evidence of normal or depressed myocardial contractility. Am J Cardiol 52:813–817

Suwa M, Hirota Y, Kawamura K (1983) Effects of nifedipine on left ventricular systolic and diastolic function in hypertrophic nonobstructive cardiomyopathy: an echocardiographic observation. J Cardiovasc Ultrasonogr 2:9–17

Wynne J. Braunwald E (1984) Hypertrophic cardiomyopathy. In: Braunwald E (ed) Heart disease. A textbook of cardiovascular medicine, 2nd edn. Saunders, Philadelphia, pp 1409–1421

Yamaguchi H, Ishimura T, Nishiyama S, Nagasaki F, Nakanishi S et al. (1979) Hypertrophic nonobstructive cardiomyopathy with giant negative T wave (apical hypertrophy): ventriculographic and echocardiographic features in 30 patients. Am J Cardiol 44:401–412

Yutani C, Imakita M. Ishibashi-Ueda H, Hatanaka K, Nagata S, Sakakibara H, Nimura Y (1985) Three autopsy cases of progression to left ventricular dilatation in patients with hypertrophic cardiomyopathy. Am Heart J 109:545–553

Subject Index

GPSR Compliance

The European Union's (EU) General Product Safety Regulation (GPSR) is a set of rules that requires consumer products to be safe and our obligations to ensure this.

If you have any concerns about our products, you can contact us on ProductSafety@springernature.com

In case Publisher is established outside the EU, the EU authorized representative is:

Springer Nature Customer Service Center GmbH
Europaplatz 3
69115 Heidelberg, Germany

Batch number: 10704713

Printed by Printforce, the Netherlands